Unlocking Longevity

The Heart Connection

A Cardiologist's Perspective

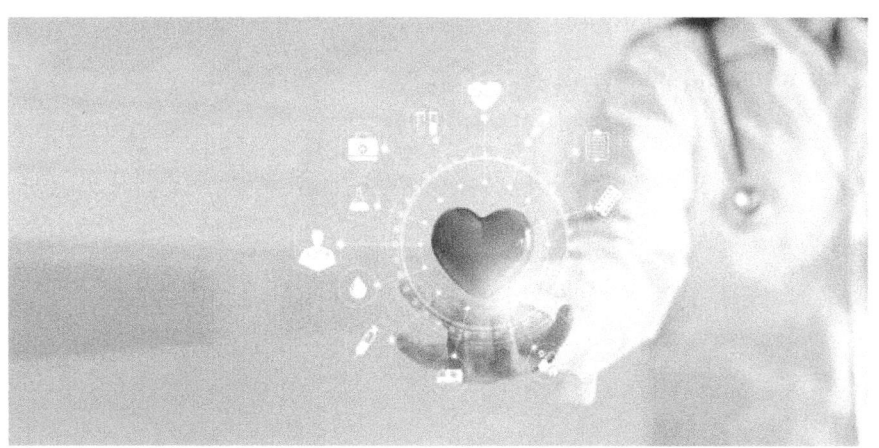

By
Peter S. Diamond, MD

Copyright © 2023 by Peter S. Diamond.

All rights reserved. No part of this publication may be reproduced, distributed, or transmitted in any form or by any means, including photocopying, recording, or other electronic or mechanical methods, without the prior written permission of the author, except in the case of brief quotations embodied in critical reviews and certain other non-commercial uses permitted by copyright law.

Ordering Information: Special discounts are available on quantity purchases by corporations, associations, as well as U.S. trade bookstores and wholesalers.

www.DreamStartersPublishing.com

Table of Contents

Introduction 5
Preface 8
Coronary Artery Disease 13
Hypertension 37
Diabetes 52
Sleep 73
Dementia 92
Preventing the Top Five Causes of Death 119
Supplements 130
Spirituality 151
The Best Diet 161
Afterword 174
Acknowledgments 179
A Note to Physicians 181
A Note to Patients 183

"Our bodies are our gardens – our wills are our gardeners."

William Shakespeare

"Before you heal someone, ask him if he's willing to give up the things that make him sick."

Hippocrates

Introduction

Authors have various and sundry reasons for writing a book. Many people want to tell a "story," while others want to share wisdom and insights garnered from various life experiences. The talented few have incredibly imaginative minds that can create a series of books that intertwine certain themes or ongoing protagonists that jump from one crisis to another with amazing durability.

My purpose is much less complex. As a physician for the last forty years, my overall life experience has been enriched by thousands of wonderful patients and a constellation of incredible colleagues in various medical specialties. Early in my career, I foolishly thought that I understood the qualities necessary to provide the best health options for my patients. These interactions have afforded me a somewhat unique opportunity to reassess and renegotiate the extraordinarily complex pathways that lead to optimum health. It is this experiential process that has prompted me to write down some insights that I hope will benefit others seeking to improve their own health.

Medicine has been the avenue for nurturing virtue in myself and in those whom I serve as a physician. I certainly did not start my career with such noble intentions. For the most part, the pathway to a medical career is quite self-centered and self-absorbing for those who choose to pursue it. The pressure and focus to be accepted to the best university and excel academically frequently requires sacrifices of time, relationships, and even self-health to qualify for medical school. Medical school acceptance rates are approximately one percent of total applicants, and acceptance only invites further self-absorption and focus until the next hurdle is encountered. Internship, residency, and fellowship training brings even more increased levels of stress that wreak havoc on sleep habits, eating habits, and emotional stability. It is not an easy road, but the rewards can be immeasurable.

Along this journey, I have found that my approach to care has oscillated from an aggressive one that depended heavily on medications and interventions to a more fundamental approach that integrates preventative and lifestyle medicine in addition to necessary medications and treatments. This has been a slow and methodical learning experience that has not been without hazard and difficulty. I have found that prescribing less while listening and teaching more has brought immeasurable rewards for both me and my patients. I have greater satisfaction knowing I am now focusing on the underlying causes of disease so prevention and true healing can occur. This approach also relies on the active participation of each patient in their own personal health, making it less autocratic and more of a mutually beneficial relationship whereby satisfaction increases for professionals and patients—when patients adhere to professionals' advice.

Sadly, the amount of time required in this new paradigm can be exhausting. In addition, a substantial number of my patients fail to adhere to my advice despite my commitment to their well-being. The doctors' "return on investment" from spending additional time on patients who aren't adhering to their recommendations can be frustrating and unrewarding. We want to be known as the "accountability office" when patients exit their appointment, but the follow-up results are quite variable. In some ways, I feel the frustration of biblical prophets whose messages were ignored. So often, my words seem to fall on deaf ears. Patients continue to eat poorly and fail to exercise, and then they wonder why they continue to spend so much time and money on medical care. Our visits become a mutual frustration session.

As a potential solution to this conundrum, I have created this book as a written educational resource through which my patients could review the available information that has guided my treatment decisions. This material could then be used for self-learning and implementation at any time. Most of the illnesses that I evaluate in my office are modifiable and potentially curable without large amounts of medication. I have come to learn that many patients are quite willing to adopt a holistic approach to healthcare that includes the use of integrative methods of healing. And as such, I now enjoy being a medication "depopulator."

Adopting this new methodology was a great learning experience for me and has encouraged me to advance the concept of discovering and treating the root causes of illness so prevention and cure are feasible. It was not easy for me initially because of my allopathic medical training, but I now recognize it as the best approach to medical care. I am very blessed and grateful to God for the ability to minister to my fellow man.

Hippocrates stated,

> *"Wherever the art of Medicine is loved, there is also a love of Humanity."*

Along this challenging but beautiful path, I have been able to shed some of my initial self-absorption as I have learned to care for others. It has been an invaluable experience in my personal development. I am deeply grateful for the opportunity.

Ultimately, this book is a labor of love for my patients. They have taught me the value of trust and caring. They have become a part of my own extended family. This is my simple gift to them. Jesus teaches that one of the greatest commandments is to "Love your neighbor as yourself" (Matthew 22:39 NIV). I believe that this book is a way of reflecting that love. It is a simple message with a profound meaning.

I pray that you enjoy the book.

Preface

I have always wanted a Range Rover. The Range Rover is a very sleek and beautiful high-performance vehicle. I live in Wisconsin, and this SUV can negotiate terrible road conditions, such as snow and sleet. It is beautifully designed on the outside with sleek angles, soft edges, and an efficient design, and it is luxurious and highly well-appointed on the inside, making the driver feel great. As an attractive car that stands out in a crowded parking lot and seems to perform challenging tasks with little effort, it has something for everyone to desire.

Despite all its qualities and benefits, the Range Rover does not list in the top fifty most researched cars on a popular automobile website. For many people, the car is too expensive to own. They cannot justify the amount of work and effort they must undertake to afford such an asset. Others likely feel that high maintenance costs will make it a challenging long-term investment. Some do not want to pursue their dream of owning such a perfect machine, and they walk away before even going for a test drive.

Does this sound familiar to you? Does the metaphor of the Range Rover bring into focus the issue that faces so many when it comes to seeking good long-term health? As a species, human beings have many similar desires. Good health and happiness are at the pinnacle of those desires for most of us. Of course, success, wealth, intelligence, and attractiveness are also high on our list. Yet without our health or happiness, our other desires seem much less important to achieve.

In His Sermon on the Mount, Jesus told the story of the wise man who built his home on a rock to avoid its being destroyed in a storm. In a similar light, we must create both a physical and a spiritual foundation that is solid and resistant to the forces of the world. I believe that sleep is one of the four components of a solid physical foundation for long-term health. The others include good nutrition, regular exercise, and avoiding toxins such as sugar and smoking.

Health is a choice. If you choose wisely, your foundation will be strong, and you will likely be well protected against the onslaught of age and disease that is always gently knocking at the door.

Most people assume that good health requires hard work, luck, or good genes. Most people are wrong. A healthy, happy, and productive life is not complicated. It does require the four "selfs" that I will discuss later in this book: self-denial, self-reliance, self-discipline, and self-sacrifice. Good health results primarily from healthy food choices, avoiding common toxins in our environment (cigarettes and trans fats are a few examples), regular exercise, good social interactions, spirituality, and a purposeful life.

Lousy food, a sedentary lifestyle, smoking, and overabundant sugar consumption have been enemies of the human body for generations. As our health becomes poorer, the pharmaceutical and device industries become richer. We are now facing a tsunami of obesity, diabetes, hypertension, and dementia. The foundation of these illnesses is inflammation. The avoidance and the treatment of inflammation should be the cornerstone of therapy, but statins, diabetic and hypertension medications, and joint replacement have become the standard of care. What we need to do is treat inflammation, but many lack the discipline and fortitude needed to combat inflammation by eating well, exercising, sleeping effectively, and avoiding smoking. Yet they are also highly effective. Society cannot complain about rising healthcare costs and tacitly ignore the responsibility that each person must take to optimize health. We must all aspire to excellent health and inspire others to do the same. Physicians alone cannot solve these issues. We must act together. Our role as doctors is perhaps better suited to a vision that was imagined so many years ago:

"The doctor of the future will give no medicine but will instruct his patients in the care of the human frame, in diet, and the cause and prevention of disease." (Thomas Edison)

While we know that's what we need, we all struggle with finding the best diet, the most beneficial supplements, and the most attractive workout gear. We spend endless hours researching the latest fads in superfoods, the best and most simple exercises for the perfect six-pack, and the healthiest grocery items. Just like the Range Rover phenomenon, we see thin and attractive models and celebrities with beautiful bodies selling these products, and we read about their excellent relationships and their newly discovered happiness. We want to have what they have. They probably drive a Range Rover too!

In the end, however, we struggle to make the meaningful health changes that we are told will help us feel and look better. We join the expensive health club, but we don't attend. We take the supplements for a while and then stop because they become "too expensive." We gain more weight, have more aches and pains, seem less happy and lose our dream of achieving good health and happiness. We start to lose sleep and take sleep aids. We develop back pain and knee pain and headaches and heartburn. We can't seem to lose weight even though we are eating less. We notice sags and belly fat, so we stop socializing because we don't like how we look. Our days are spent with our computer and television. Our lives become mundane and predictable, and our true happiness slowly slips away to sadness and depression. Our interpersonal problems erode our spouses, friends, and children. We release our dreams and convince ourselves that nothing will help. We deny ourselves the essential hope necessary to find the strength to change our habits and lifestyle. We convince ourselves that we are metabolically different because any food seems to make us gain weight.

If any or all of these things sound familiar to you, be assured of two things: You are not alone, and there is hope that you can still change and feel much better. Matthew Kelly is a spiritual writer who describes a fascinating weakness we as human beings seem to have in common: *Resisting Happiness*. In his acclaimed book that I highly recommend you read (titled the same), he explains the features of this phenomenon. What he identifies and describes cannot be understated: God created us to be happy. In many ways, we cannot or will not accept this tenet. And so, if we do not believe in God, we cannot understand and comprehend the concept that He created us to live a happy and fulfilled life. This includes good health.

In Kelly's words,

"God wants you to be happy even more than you want it yourself. It is time to stop resisting happiness. It's time to slay resistance."

For over forty years, I have cared for patients who have a constellation of severe and ongoing health problems. Usually, these medical issues do not occur in isolation. Diabetes, hypertension, lipid disorders, and orthopedic issues tend to join forces in one body at the same time. As a cardiologist, I treat multiple interrelated issues to avoid future medical catastrophes such as heart attacks, strokes, kidney failure, or bypass surgery. I must confess that in many ways, I fail my patients because I cannot seem to motivate them to lose weight, start the exercise program, take the correct supplements, or upgrade their spiritual and social lives to avoid the medical pitfalls that most likely await them. As much as patients suffer from the ravages and consequences of their diseases, physicians also suffer, albeit differently.

The doctor-patient relationship can be a unique, precious, and gratifying experience for physicians. In many ways, we invite you into our extended family as we "visit" together every few weeks or months. Contrary to the typical business model of finding ways to establish a return business sector, most good physicians desire good health and long, happy lives for their "customers" so that they don't need to return except for an occasional wellness evaluation.

Doctors are compassionate human beings who do not enjoy our fellow man's suffering. In many ways, love for others and a strong desire for their good health and happiness are the foundation of my relationship with my patients. In the Gospel of Mark (1:40–45 NIV), a leper knelt before Jesus and implored Him, saying, "If you are willing, you can make me clean." Jesus, the preeminent healer and model of all physicians, responded in this way: "Moved with pity, He stretched out his hand, touched him and said to him, I do will it. Be made clean." At that moment, the leper was cured. I want my patients to know that I am moved by empathy for them. Like Jesus, I desire for them to be healed. I also know that I am only a humble servant of Christ and do not have His healing powers. Despite my limitations, I want to find a better, more effective, and more successful way to help my patients become healed. This is the reason for this book. I know that the life of that leper was changed radically for good. And just like him, true happiness and good health await anyone that seeks help and is genuinely open to change.

Just as that Range Rover embodies all the elements that would make it an excellent fit for all of us, good health can be a reality for all of us. We must remind ourselves that we can make our exterior design sleek and attractive and our "interior" design very functional and clean with the proper nutrition and supplementation. We must dream again and be willing to work for what we want and desire: good health and happiness. With these two powerful assets, we will be capable of negotiating all of life's bumpy roads as we travel on this beautiful journey of life.

Chapter 1

Coronary Artery Disease

July 1, 1983, was an exciting and memorable Friday for me. I had completed my cardiology fellowship one week earlier and was starting my first day in a group practice in Oak Lawn, Illinois. I was trained as both an invasive and noninvasive cardiologist to perform most of the cardiac testing available at that time, including angiograms of patients' coronary arteries. At that time, cardiologists recognized that coronary artery disease was caused when cholesterol buildup in the heart arteries caused blockages that restricted blood flow through the involved vessel. We also knew that sudden occlusion (heart attack) was caused by clot formation within the artery that stopped flow within the vessel. In essence, the prevalent disease that I was treating was cholesterol. Smoking, high blood pressure, and diabetes were important subplots in this process, but cholesterol was the enemy.

I was on call on my very first day in practice. My first patient, Bob, had developed chest pain after golfing with his wife.

He was active and otherwise healthy, with only mild newly diagnosed diabetes. When I arrived in the emergency room to see him, he was acutely ill and amid a heart attack. At that time, we did not perform emergency angiograms for opening arteries and placing stents. Studies at that time had shown the efficacy of clot-busting drugs, but my hospital had never used these agents. Fortunately, streptokinase, one of these drugs, was available in the hospital pharmacy, and I coaxed the emergency room doctors and nurses to try this new agent. I remained at the patient's bedside over the next several hours. Approximately one hour after starting this infusion, his pain resolved, and his EKG markedly improved. We all breathed easier until his heart suddenly stopped. Fortunately, we were prepared for this possibility, and one shock restored his heart rhythm to normal. The remainder of his hospitalization was uneventful, and he was discharged home several days later.

What was intriguing to me during that hospitalization was that Bob's cholesterol was normal. Over the next twenty-five years, I had the pleasure of caring for Bob. He did not smoke, and his blood pressure was always perfect, and he didn't have a family history of heart disease. However, he had a poor, uncontrolled diet, and his diabetes soon required two drugs. Despite his unremarkable cholesterol numbers, he developed progressive symptoms of chest discomfort, and he was found to have severe three-vessel coronary artery disease within the next few years. He required coronary bypass surgery to alleviate the chest pain that was preventing him from playing his beloved game of golf with his wife. He began a statin drug in 1987 when these new "miracle" cures first became available. Despite his low cholesterol numbers, he continued to have progressive coronary artery disease, and he suffered two more heart attacks and required subsequent stent placement. He was forced to give up golf, and his activity level dropped. He was never able to change his diet and was convinced that his food choices were not pertinent to his heart disease.

Bob's story reflects the mindset toward coronary artery disease (CAD) that has been present for several decades in the medical community. Cholesterol buildup was seen as the biggest issue, and so lowering patients' cholesterol levels was the goal for most physicians. To a large extent, this mindset persists today in both the medical community and the population at large. This thought process has caused the pharmaceutical and food industries to thrive with cholesterol-lowering strategies. The idea that other causes of CAD could have a role in this often-fatal disease has been minimized or ignored.

In addition, the statin story's dark side is the pharmaceutical industry's incredible role in marketing and promoting their products under dubious scientific methodology. More disdainful to me, however, is the active participation of "respected" researchers in propagating some misleading critical benefits of statin use. An enormous problem has evolved regarding conflict of interest between the pharmaceutical and device companies and physicians that appears to be primarily linked to financial rewards. I am particularly disheartened by the role of doctors in this deceitful process because they are already highly compensated professionals. Greed and manipulation are human weaknesses that are not isolated to medicine. Still, it must be seen as immoral when this behavior impacts individual health and well-being.

Over the past twenty years, a growing body of laboratory and human studies has shed more light on the role inflammation plays in the development of vascular disease in general and CAD specifically. Not only is it a factor with CAD, but inflammation plays a role in diseases of the GI tract, the musculoskeletal system, and many other organ systems. Although cholesterol factors into the development of CAD, the primary culprit appears to be inflammation. Not treating this inflammation is much like a homeowner who fails to recognize and treat a termite problem. Eventually, the house falls apart after recurrent leaks and other structural issues. Despite this valuable scientific contribution to our knowledge of CAD, cholesterol treatment remains the big target of therapy, while inflammation is primarily ignored and minimized. This error is critical in recognizing why heart disease remains the number one killer of men and women today.

    We have long been aware of the so-called traditional risk factors for CAD: advancing age, diabetes, hypertension, smoking, high cholesterol, male sex, and family history of heart disease. In addition, physical inactivity has been recognized as an additional risk for CAD. Despite these risks, several nontraditional risk factors may play a significant, if not more important, role. A 2018 update from the American College of Cardiology acknowledges that there is currently no one proven way to eliminate risk of cardiovascular disease. However, applying traditional risk factors alone ignores the increased risk in lower-socioeconomic groups, patients with inflammatory conditions such as rheumatoid arthritis, patients with kidney disease, and specific at-risk racial and ethnic populations. Insulin resistance—and especially metabolic syndrome—are highly associated with CAD but are not included in current screening formulas. Metabolic syndrome is a constellation of risk factors associated with a significantly enhanced risk of developing CAD and other forms of vascular disease. These risks include hypertension, elevated triglycerides, low HDL level, abdominal obesity, and elevated blood sugar. Almost two-thirds of patients presenting with an acute myocardial infarction will have clinical evidence of metabolic syndrome and, sadly, about 30 percent of the US population qualifies for it.

We must recognize that many factors place us at risk for CAD. Fooling ourselves into believing it is all about cholesterol levels distracts us from a prevention strategy that focuses on reducing inflammation.

Inflammation

Atherosclerosis, or hardening of the arteries, primarily affects large- and medium-sized arteries in the human body, including the coronary arteries that supply the heart with nutrient-rich blood. Think of the coronary artery as a hollow, flexible tube. The innermost lining of this tube comprises a single layer of cells that resembles a cobblestone street. It is a porous lining that allows nutrients and other blood components, including LDL cholesterol (frequently referred to as "bad" cholesterol) particles, to move through and pass deeper into the arterial wall. This cell layer also produces chemical substances that relax or constrict the arteries, directly affecting their size. In normal, noninflammatory conditions, there is a stable interplay between these chemical substances that allows for appropriate constriction and dilation of the arterial wall.

However, when inflammatory conditions provoked by diabetes, hypertension, poor dietary intake, and other factors occur, there is an imbalance in the production of these substances. This ultimately leads to constriction and instability of the arterial lining. As a consequence, the arterial lining produces a substance that makes it "sticky," which, in turn, attracts immune cells known as lymphocytes. Furthermore, free radicals, which are overproduced in inflammatory conditions, oxidize LDL particles, and make them much more dangerous. When the "cobblestone" arterial lining becomes inflamed, the "cobblestones" separate from each other to some degree. As a result, the oxidized LDL particles can slip between the gaps in the cells and get trapped in the inner layers of the arterial wall. The lymphocytes follow and engulf the oxidized LDL, which leads to the release of more chemicals that cause the process to snowball. The mix of cells eventually forms foam cells, smooth muscle cells are attracted to join in, and the atherosclerotic plaque matures. If this interplay continues long term, the size of the plaque will grow.

Interestingly, the volume of plaque does not initially cause the narrowing of the artery—this is because of the entire arterial wall's elasticity—rather the outermost layer of the artery stretches to accommodate the increased mass within the diseased arterial segment. That is why diseased coronary arteries are larger in total diameter than standard segments. Eventually, the outermost layer can expand no further, and the inner portion of the artery begins to narrow.

If the process is left unabated, the pressure from the expanding soft plaque places tension on the artery's thin and fragile innermost lining. If this layer becomes overwhelmed, it will tear, and the "volcano effect" releases materials that attract platelets and clotting factors. This leads to an acute increase in overall plaque size, primarily composed of clotting elements. If the formed clot becomes large enough, it will block the artery and lead to an acute heart attack, and even smaller clots usually lead to symptoms of acute chest pain or other complaints characteristic of an impending heart attack. At this critical stage, antiplatelet medications such as aspirin and anticoagulation therapy such as heparin or Lovenox can be very effective in stopping or slowing acute clot formation.

Based on this description of plaque formation, cholesterol treatment should be the secondary, not primary, focus of treating CAD. Inflammation is the foundation of other vascular diseases as well, including hypertension. Despite this well-known scientific premise, cholesterol-lowering strategies receive excessive focus and financial backing. Yet, cholesterol-lowering drugs (primarily statins) have never consistently shown a significant decrease in death from cardiovascular causes, despite an overwhelming amount of marketing and medical writings. This disturbing concept was initially challenging for me to accept after a long career treating patients with various degrees of CAD. While I will cover cholesterol treatment in a subsequent chapter, I would like to focus a limited time on the causes of atherosclerosis. To better understand this term, atherosclerosis is a degenerative process in all arteries that is caused by inflammation and subsequent cholesterol and plaque development. CAD is a byproduct of progressive atherosclerosis, much like rust is a byproduct of environmental oxidation.

As a physician, it is far easier to prescribe a statin drug for high cholesterol than it is to spend time reviewing the tremendous benefits of an anti-inflammatory diet and an effective exercise program. It is much easier for patients to take a pill than to begin a more restrictive dietary regimen. Taking medicine daily falsely convinces us that the benefits of statin and blood pressure pills overcome our natural reluctance to perform daily exercise. The supplement industry also benefits from this mindset, but an individual can never out-supplement a poor diet or lack of exercise. A focused lifestyle change is imperative to reduce the long-term risk of CAD. Otherwise, we doom ourselves and our bodies to a life of disease and suffering. Although it may be challenging, we have this beautiful opportunity to avoid this suffering and begin to enjoy a life of health and happiness.

Diagnosing and Treating CAD in the Office

As a cardiologist, I have a large armamentarium of testing tools to assess the presence or absence of coronary artery disease. My approach to diagnosis and treatment may seem somewhat different than many within my Cardiology community. If the origin of this disease is inflammatory, assessing inflammation and other inflammatory-related factors, such as insulin resistance, is the crux of my initial assessment. During my initial consultation with a new patient, I inquire about lifestyle factors such as diet and exercise habits. I also review their body size and shape. Sadly, most patients I see for cardiovascular evaluation are overweight, and a substantial percentage meet the criteria for obesity. The BMI is a calculation utilizing body weight related to height and serves as a valuable tool for informing and guiding patients about their actual body size. I cannot tell you how many times patients have told me that their elevated BMI is related to the fact that they are "big-boned." I gently remind them that their bones are not made of lead, and the protruding gut likely contributes to their increased weight!

The presence of other illnesses or inflammatory conditions can frequently be a clue to my patients' underlying risk for CAD. For instance, gingival disease and poor dentition are markers for inflammation and are associated with a higher risk of CAD. Good oral hygiene and avoidance of smoking can have a beneficial effect on dental care. Still, healthy diets and regular exercise improve dental health and lower the risk of periodontal disease. Good oral hygiene does not prevent heart disease, but simply opening your mouth may provide a window into your underlying state of inflammation.

I see many patients who have both CAD and joint disease. I am amazed at the number of patients who have already undergone joint replacement at a young age. Although some are obese, many patients are not grossly overweight. A common association seems to be the presence of diabetes or Metabolic Syndrome. I suspect that underlying inflammation is the primary culprit. These individuals often have back pain and nonspecific muscle discomfort as other indicators of inflammation. In addition, these musculoskeletal issues frequently become an excuse for avoiding exercise, even when it is well-known that frequent low-level exercise can significantly benefit overall joint health and maintenance of muscle mass. I remind my recalcitrant patients that regular aerobic training and weightlifting a few days a week will accrue great long-term benefits on overall joint and cardiovascular health. It is also likely that their aches and pains will lessen as they accrue the anti-inflammatory benefits of these activities.

As part of an initial assessment for CAD, I utilize elevated inflammatory markers as a guidepost for treatment. High-sensitivity CRP (hs-CRP) is a valuable tool for me. An advanced lipid profile is also beneficial in some patients because it provides more quantitative evidence of cholesterol particle numbers. A standard cholesterol panel can provide very helpful information. I focus less on LDL and total cholesterol levels and target the triglyceride/HDL (Tri/HDL) ratio. An ideal ratio is 2:1 or less. An elevated Tri/HDL ratio of 4:1 is a valuable predictor of risk for future cardiac events such as heart attacks and strokes. A high triglyceride/HDL ratio is also a good indicator of insulin resistance. Metabolic Syndrome is almost always present when these abnormalities are associated with increased body weight, belt size, and blood sugar. This syndrome should be considered a severe and potentially ominous entity, as approximately two-thirds of patients with acute heart attacks will have this abnormal profile. I will often order a glycohemoglobin level to ascertain if diabetes is present. A fasting insulin level is also very helpful to determine if insulin resistance may be present.

Yes. I consider Metabolic Syndrome an "illness" because it is associated with a high risk of diffuse vascular disease and CAD. If untreated or minimized as a medical condition, future health will be negatively affected, and cardiovascular morbidity and mortality will be significantly increased. The good news is that optimizing diet and regular exercise can dramatically reduce the complications of this illness. The bad news is that most patients shrug their shoulders and accept their fate because they are unwilling to change their habits.

Exercise testing is a widespread and likely overused screening tool for CAD. Various cardiac stress tests involve active and passive cardiovascular system stimulation. A modified standard treadmill is used per a pre-set protocol to gradually increase exercise intensity in patients who can tolerate rigorous activity. In patients who have activity limitations or orthopedic or neurological issues, medications can be infused by IV access. Dobutamine and Adenosine-analogs are common agents that I use. The IV studies usually incorporate an additional imaging modality such as echocardiography or nuclear imaging. I strongly favor echocardiography over any nuclear study because of the radiation risk associated with nuclear imaging. In almost all instances, echocardiography can supplant nuclear imaging when an experienced reading cardiologist performs the interpretation. I am particularly discouraged by the large number of nuclear studies performed on younger patients, especially women of childbearing age. To me, this is highly unnecessary and irresponsible, and it places the patient at undue long-term risk if exposed to a lifetime of imaging.

    Sensitivity and specificity are essential terms to understand when attempting to understand stress testing and its limited value in screening for CAD. In simple terms, sensitivity reflects a test's capacity to detect disease when it is truly present. On the other hand, specificity reveals the ability to exclude illness when it is truly absent. In the ideal world of cardiovascular disease testing, we would have a test with 100% accuracy in detecting CAD (high sensitivity) and a 100% capacity to exclude CAD (high specificity). A normal test would genuinely mean that no significant disease is present. Unfortunately, stress imaging studies are not the perfect tool. In my career, I have seen many studies that are poor predictors of disease presence. There appear to be many false positive tests that frequently require further testing. There is also a smaller but significant number of studies that are falsely negative and can provide false confidence regarding cardiovascular risk and discourage prevention strategies. In the best circumstances, stress nuclear and stress echocardiography studies have a sensitivity of 80-85%, but this highly depends on the lab and the reading physician. Stress testing has a sensitivity of perhaps 70%, but many other variables can affect results, including duration of exercise, peak heart rate achieved, and baseline EKG features.

I generally do not use stress testing as a random screening tool for CAD anymore unless I have a sedentary patient with multiple risk factors planning to begin a regular vigorous exercise program. In my patients with chest pain and risk factors for CAD, stress testing is an excellent tool for assessing symptoms and reassuring lower-risk patients that it is acceptable to resume or begin an exercise regimen. I reserve stress echocardiography for patients at intermediate risk for CAD with chest pain or new complaints of shortness of breath. I also find stress echocardiography to be a valuable tool for my patients with mitral valve prolapse or pre-existing EKG abnormalities because of the higher incidence of false positive EKG changes during exercise. I decide on a medical infusion study versus a walking stress test during my initial cardiac assessment. I watch patient movement and walking skills and can usually discriminate which patients need a "chemical" stress study.

I can offer some advice about stress testing in the presence of known CAD. If you are a patient with a previous coronary bypass or stent (or if you have known non-critical CAD), your cardiologist may advise you to get regular stress testing. In the absence of new or progressive cardiac symptoms, there is rarely an indication to perform these studies. Screening for advanced disease or early detection is often the reason for these unnecessary exams. Your cardiologist may insist on these studies with vague reasoning and explanations. Still, best practice guidelines do not support this approach, and false positive studies in asymptomatic patients often lead to more risky testing, such as coronary angiography. Be especially wary if your doctor insists the investigation be performed only in their office. It may well be a financial incentive that is driving this recommendation.

Coronary Calcium Screening (CCS) has been available for many years and can help screen high-risk individuals. This screening study is painless (no needles or injections) and allows for the quantification of calcification within the inner lining of the coronary arteries. Values are age-dependent and generally increase with age. The study will provide an absolute calcium score and measure everyone's Calcium score relative to age and sex distribution. In my practice, I use the investigation only on patients at least 40 years old (men) or 45-50 in women. The predictive value of this study is much less valuable in younger patients. The study involves short-term radiation exposure performed using a CT scanner. Recent studies suggest that the average low-level radiation (1.0mSv) received is equivalent to 10 chest X-rays. Compared to our daily radiation exposure, this is the equivalent of 1 year of natural background radiation and cannot be considered insignificant.

The use of CCS has been somewhat controversial in Cardiology circles. Still, it serves a limited but valuable role in assessing chest pain in intermediate-risk patients. It also can eliminate the need for statin therapy in many patients with elevated cholesterol who have a low or 0 score. This concept is critical to understand because many doctors will insist on statin therapy for elevated cholesterol even when the Calcium score is 0. I will address this issue in another chapter, but high cholesterol does not always indicate the presence of underlying CAD. I also find that an abnormally elevated CCS can serve as a motivational tool for high-risk patients with poor insight into their long-term health risks. One additional blood test that I recommend in those individuals with elevated coronary calcium is Lp(a). This blood test is a screening tool for higher-risk patients with a family history of CAD and elevation of the Coronary Calcium Score. It is a genetic marker associated with an increased risk of CAD. Some eminent cardiologists suggest screening for elevated Lp(a) in most individuals, and I cannot disagree with this approach.

The most recent study directly addresses calcium scoring, and statin therapy (JACC Nov 2018) suggests a significant benefit for patients with a coronary calcium score of greater than 100. However, statistically, the number needed to treat (NNT) was 12 to see a reduction in stroke, heart attack, or death from cardiovascular disease in 1 patient. Taken another way, 11 of 12 treated patients with a calcium score greater than 100 gain no long-term benefit from statin therapy. Shared decision-making is essential in such circumstances because treatment will likely be a lifetime commitment, and statins will further augment the calcium scores if future scoring studies are undertaken.

The refinement of CT scanning has allowed for much better imaging of the coronary arteries over the past several years. The biggest obstacle with this assessment of coronary artery disease in the past was the heart's constant motion, which made optimized image acquisition very difficult because of artifactual distortion. Today's CT scanners have much better "shutter speeds" that allow for excellent opacification of the coronary arteries with minimal image loss. In addition, the recent acquisition of flow reserve measurements to assess the true functional significance of a narrowed segment has further validated this modality. Still, it must be used in very select patients whose stress testing results have been non-diagnostic, and the likelihood of disease is not significant enough to warrant an invasive angiogram. This study can also be used for patients with primary valvular heart problems awaiting surgical treatment. CT imaging can replace standard angiograms in lower-risk patients and significantly lower cost and risk. The primary negative aspect of this testing is related to radiation exposure. In addition, if significant symptomatic disease within the coronary arteries is identified, a formal coronary angiogram may be necessary to consider angioplasty and stunting.

Advances in CT technology continue to allow for valuable information in high-risk patients. Artificial intelligence (AI) is playing a role in this diagnostic field. AI-assisted imaging (Coronary Computed Tomography Angiography (CCTA) is an exciting new tool that can assess plaque burden within each coronary artery and determine the stability of each plaque. Unstable plaques are more dangerous. Aggressive treatment options and lowered risk are excellent benefits of this type of study. Unfortunately, insurance coverage for this new advancement is not guaranteed at the time of this writing.

      The gold standard for assessing symptomatic CAD remains cardiac catheterization. We, as cardiologists, frequently use the terms cardiac catheterization and coronary angiography interchangeably, but "catheterization" primarily means introducing a catheter into the heart. Coronary angiography means dye injection in the coronary arteries to look for blockages. Although the risk of this procedure is low, it is not without its potential risks and complications. As a former interventional cardiologist, I was amazed at the cavalier attitude of non-invasive cardiologists and non-cardiac physicians towards this procedure. Many physicians think this is a simple procedure like cleaning your teeth. As a physician who has lost some years of my life sweating the challenges of acutely ill patients in the catheterization laboratory, I can assure you that this procedure has some real risks. I generally inform patients that there is a 1% chance of a heart attack and a .01% chance of death. Shared decision-making is essential because there is also a minimal but real risk of stroke, arterial injury, and kidney damage. I have been very privileged to work with some of the best men and women who perform these interventional procedures, and we have all faced the heartbreak of a complication in the lab. I have always said that if I knew who would suffer a difficulty, I would never perform the procedure on that patient. Unfortunately, we don't possess that clairvoyance. We must also acknowledge that the medical profession remains an inexact science and that the potential for errors or incorrect judgments will always exist. Therefore, any decision to proceed with this invasive procedure must be seriously weighed against the risks and benefits of obtaining the desired information from this study.

Cardiac MRI has recently evolved as a helpful tool in diagnosing some forms of heart disease. It is particularly valuable in assessing left ventricular muscle abnormalities (Cardiomyopathy) and beneficial for valvular issues and some congenital heart abnormalities. It does not expose the patient to harmful radiation, but it is a very long and loud procedure that frequently requires injecting a particular imaging contrast agent. I believe cardiac MRI has excellent future potential in cardiac imaging. Still, it is perhaps too time-intensive and costly to replace other imaging modalities. It also requires a great deal of patience on the part of the patient, and it is not currently capable of accurately assessing the coronary artery tree optimally.

Once a diagnosis is established, each patient must decide their desired treatment pathway. A myriad of medications and procedures are currently available for the treatment of both symptomatic and asymptomatic CAD. Unfortunately, these options may not be adequately explained by healthcare professionals, and patients may be confused about risks and benefits. Therefore, everyone must explore and educate themselves before proceeding with more aggressive treatment options. As a matter of explanation, primary prevention in cardiology is a treatment that focuses on preventing disease before it occurs. Secondary prevention is a treatment approach for patients who already have established or identified disease.

Below are some of the treatment options available today:

- Aspirin. While this used to be one of the most prescribed medications for asymptomatic CAD, it has now been established that aspirin likely has no beneficial role in the

primary prevention of heart attacks in patients at risk. Furthermore, aspirin has small but significant side effects, including bleeding and stomach irritation. If you have never had a heart attack, a stent, or open-heart surgery for bypass or valve replacement, you do not need to take aspirin.
- Statin therapy is more controversial in the primary treatment of CAD and, perhaps, secondary prevention. Statin therapy has been widely touted as an excellent prevention tool in patients with elevated cholesterol and other related risk factors. The conventional thinking in the cardiovascular community for the past few decades was that the data regarding the benefits of statins in both groups were settled and inarguable. However, the actual benefits are much smaller than most doctors and patients think, as a critical and open-minded review of the literature shows. Suffice it to say, statin benefits have been markedly overhyped, and the side effects are likely more significant than aspirin.
- Beta-blockers and nitrate therapy remain at the forefront of treatment for patients with symptomatic CAD. They alleviate the symptoms of chest pain that can accompany severe artery blockage. In addition, certain beta-blockers have a beneficial role in prolonging survival in patients who have suffered a heart attack.
- Calcium channel blockers can also be effective, especially when a spasm of the coronary artery is suspected. Add-on drugs can play a limited role in some patients with chest pain caused by CAD, but the benefits are negligible.
- Natural supplements have been successful for some patients with chest discomfort. Still, drug interactions and side effects can occur, and they should be used under physician advisement. Vitamin C may play a unique role in the underlying treatment of cholesterol deposition within the

artery, but it remains controversial. Vitamin K2 may also benefit patients with significant coronary calcification.

Interventional Treatment of CAD

On September 16, 1977, German cardiologist Andreas Gruentzig performed the first angioplasty of a coronary artery in Switzerland. This momentous event led to a new treatment paradigm for symptomatic CAD. In my experience, coronary angioplasty (balloon expansion of the blocked artery) and coronary stenting (balloon and stent placement within the narrowed artery) have been a remarkable and lifesaving advance in the field of cardiology, but they are also markedly overutilized in our current era of advanced medical care. In this procedure, a small flexible wire is placed in the narrowed segment of an artery, and an expandable balloon is inflated to open the area of blockage. Most often, a second balloon with a small metal cylinder called a stent is then positioned into the newly opened area, and the stent is embedded into the arterial wall. If properly placed, the stent will never move or migrate. Over time, new tissue grows over the stent to remodel the arterial segment into a regular-sized opening.

Many of us in the interventional world have the "oculostenotic" reflex. The eye (oculus) sees a narrowing (stenosis) and feels a strong need to fix it. We used to think we were providing our patients an excellent service with our treatments, but research lagged behind the practice. As it turns out, like many things in medicine, a counterintuitive process occurred in patients who were not having acute heart attacks or unstable chest pain: stents were not the little lifesaving devices we thought they were. We were doing things the patient did not necessarily need because we could see the results and follow them as they seemed to improve. We failed to realize that a large majority of these patients were on medical treatments that were woefully inadequate. Medical treatment was not an "option" because a tight blockage existed. We thought this process to be an easily understandable cause-and-effect relationship. That was true until science started to catch up.

We were opening arteries with stents in patients who did not have symptoms, thinking that if we performed the procedure, we would be helping to divert problems down the line. This is called the "clogged pipe theory." We intuitively thought the pipe would eventually close off the flow and cause problems, so we tried to be proactive in treatment. We were not looking at the underlying causes of the clogged pipe and did not give enough attention to this process with our medical treatment. We now know that adjusting lifestyle, optimizing medications, and avoiding stents lead to the same result **without** the stent procedure. We likely did many unneeded procedures, but we didn't know better.

In April 2007, an important and transformative study published in the *New England Journal of Medicine* (COURAGE Trial) revealed that angioplasty and stenting did not improve survival and did not reduce the risk of heart attack or other major cardiac events when compared to medical therapy in symptomatic patients with documented severe CAD. Medical therapy, broadly termed, uses targeted medications, like statins and blood pressure medications (aspirin), and lifestyle changes that encourage smoking cessation, exercise, and dietary changes. Medically treated patients did not receive stents or surgery. This study was critically important in its final assessment. It revealed that patients with symptomatic CAD (chest pain or its equivalent) who also had an abnormal stress test and a severe blockage (70 percent or greater of at least one coronary artery) could be safely treated with medication instead of angioplasty or bypass surgery. Furthermore, this approach was not associated with a significantly increased risk of heart attack, death, or stroke.

This study threw everybody into a tizzy. How could this be true? Several subsequent studies (ORBITA trial, ISCHEMIA Trial) confirmed these results and significantly challenged the overall treatment of documented CAD. Unfortunately, not all physicians and cardiologists have accepted it. My personal experience in patient care suggests that many cardiologists still treat patients aggressively with cardiac catheterization and stent placement without a fair trial of medical therapy. The reasons are many, but it has been hard for physicians to accept the counterintuitive results of studies that challenge accepted practice patterns. Nineteenth-century Hungarian physician Ignaz Semmelweis was a notable victim of this circumstance when he discovered that handwashing dramatically lowered the risk of infection in maternity wards. Despite this finding, fellow physicians mocked and ignored him, and the practice was primarily abandoned despite its clear benefits. To this day, careful hand hygiene techniques are appropriately utilized by healthcare workers only about 50 percent of the time, despite the clear benefits for reduced disease transmission.

Healthy Habits that Lead to Healing and Prevention of CAD

A historical evaluation of mortality trends in cardiovascular disease is very revealing. Deaths from CAD reached a pinnacle in the 1960s, when up to one-third of all deaths were attributable to heart disease. As the dangers of smoking became known and public smoking subsequently declined, so did CAD-related deaths. The advent of other interventions, such as ICU units, coronary bypass surgery, and more aggressive blood pressure control, appeared to save even more lives. Still, prevention of CAD was revealed to contribute approximately 50 percent of the mortality reduction. This mortality reduction continued for the next forty years as more and more treatment options developed, including medications and stent treatment for acute heart attacks. Still, statin use may have improved mortality by only 3–4 percent.

Recently, more concerning data suggested that this downward trend in deaths from CAD is slowing, perhaps even reversing. Much of this concern revolves around the explosion of childhood and adult obesity and a significant increase in type 1 and 2 diabetes. The development of novel treatment options for CAD has also slowed precipitously. Unfortunately, a commitment to risk factor reduction has waned in addition to the factors already mentioned. For example, the PURE study assessed the adoption of three crucial lifestyle modification strategies (smoking cessation, healthy diet adoption, and regular exercise) in patients who had suffered a heart attack or stroke. Only 4 percent of these patients adopted all three strategies even with full knowledge of their diagnosis and prognosis.

This is utterly unacceptable if we are to change the trajectory of this disease and the financial costs incurred. For reference purposes, the injectable cholesterol-lowering drug evolocumab will reduce cardiac events by about 1.5 percent over time but at a yearly fee of $6,000. The average cost of a healthy organic diet for that same individual is $350 a month for an annual cost of $4,200 and a risk reduction of 20–30 percent. It should be abundantly clear that lifestyle is cost-effective and much better for long-term cardiovascular health. We all must share the responsibility of being good stewards of our healthcare dollars and our future collective well-being.

So, where does this lead us today as we move forward on the spectrum of CAD treatment? The initial approach must always be directed toward prevention. Healthy eating habits, regular exercise, and smoking avoidance are essential. Modest calorie restriction has been shown to improve survival. The CALERIE trial revealed improved immune and metabolic parameters in patients who restricted their calories by 10–12 percent. Optimization of blood lipids and blood pressure can significantly reduce the progression of patients with established CAD. Blood sugar optimization can benefit multiple organ systems, including the heart, brain, and kidneys.

Healthy fat intake and increased protein intake indirectly diminish the progression of CAD. Stress reduction and good sleep are also very important.

Medical therapy for symptomatic and asymptomatic CAD should be the initial approach unless there is clear evidence of significant disease within the left main coronary artery. The SCOT-HEART trial recently identified the value of noninvasive imaging in identifying higher- and lower-risk groups to risk-stratify patients and begin earlier medical therapy. Provided the patient has insurance coverage, the physician properly applies strategies based on the results, and these imaging procedures are widely implemented, the disease could be detected earlier, allowing for prevention with aggressive lifestyle changes that would significantly improve patient longevity.

While procedures can be done in a doctor's office after detection, the essential treatment for those with CAD is making lifestyle adjustments by optimizing diet and engaging in regular exercise. These lifestyle changes reduce inflammation, and as I noted at the beginning of this chapter, CAD, like many other disease processes, is primarily inflammatory. Oxidative stress and inflammation of the inner lining of the coronary artery will promote plaque formation. Plaque stabilization and potential plaque regression can be achieved with an anti-inflammatory diet that includes plants, fish oil sources, and limited amounts of animal proteins. Red meat is not the enemy of heart disease when used reasonably. Eating unprocessed meat a few days a week can provide clear nutritional benefits.

The real culprits are refined starches, simple carbohydrates, and processed foods, which quickly spike blood sugar levels in a way that leads to an inflammatory response. Bad foods also injure the thin gut membrane and allow the diffusion of toxins into the bloodstream that provoke an inflammatory response. Fast food is the fast track to bad health, but we are surrounded by lousy food options throughout our day. Science shows that healthy diets that utilize whole foods, healthy fats, and limited animal proteins can diminish overall inflammation. Gut health is critically important in this inflammatory axis of health and disease, and it behooves us all to understand why.

Regular low- to moderate-exercise habits can also significantly impact overall cardiovascular risk. I encourage my patients with CAD to take the LSD approach: long slow distance. Everyone would benefit by taking even fifteen minutes a day to walk, jog, swim, or bike. A recent study from the Cleveland Clinic revealed that higher levels of exercise performance on a supervised treadmill translated into a significant benefit in long-term survival, with those who achieved the highest level of performance enjoying a 90 percent improvement in survival compared to those individuals who performed at a poor level of exercise. No pill can promise this type of benefit!

Weight loss and exercise can dramatically benefit overall well-being, but their more significant value is related to the impact on hypertension, diabetes, and cholesterol values. Obesity is an epidemic in the western world, and its consequences will likely be devastating to world health. Losing as few as ten to fifteen pounds, coupled with regular low to moderate exercise, can dramatically impact blood pressure, blood sugar, and biomarkers of inflammation.

Essentially, what we eat and how we move will determine our longevity and happiness. The good news is that these lifestyle changes can dramatically reduce the complications of this illness. The bad news is that most patients shrug their shoulders and accept their fate because they are unwilling to change their habits. This willingness to engage in unhealthy lifestyle choices makes me feel inadequate in treating my patients because my motivational discussions seem to fall on deaf ears. Please understand my frustration. My patients almost always seem to leave the office with renewed purpose and a commitment to change, but their willpower and motivation wane over time. I frequently remind my heart bypass patients that as the visible incision from coronary bypass surgery begins to fade, so too may their commitment to a renewed set of lifestyle priorities start to falter. It takes hard work every day to stay healthy.

Just as a recovering alcoholic needs to take abstinence one day at a time, so must we renew our decisions to exercise and make healthy food choices. In addition, we must seek the assistance of our spouse, our extended family, and our friends to make things work. A "community" committed to serious lifestyle change and healthy habits will enjoy excellent health and happy longevity. Dan Buettner reveals clear evidence of this phenomenon in his bestselling book *The Blue Zones*. The Blue Zones Project is a beautiful beacon to identify those variables that can lead to a long, productive, healthy, and happy life. It provides a road map for each of us to achieve optimum health and true happiness. My mantra is simple: learn the simple rules that lead to joy and prioritize these rules in our lives.

<u>Takeaways</u>

1. CAD is an inflammatory process with multiple causes.
2. Cholesterol is more of a passenger than a driver of CAD, and indiscriminate cholesterol reduction is ineffective or not warranted in many patients.
3. Reduction in inflammation through lifestyle adjustments can significantly benefit survival and longevity.
4. Environmental factors play a major role in CAD development.
5. Many tests are available to diagnose CAD but are frequently overused, and the results can be misleading. Questionable results can lead to more expensive and unnecessary testing.
6. Aggressive treatment options, including stents and coronary bypass, can be effective and lifesaving. Still, medical therapy can frequently provide the same benefit in terms of quality of

life and long-term survival.
7. Treating underlying metabolic diseases through healthy lifestyle adjustments may offer one of the most effective treatments to reduce the burden of CAD.

Chapter 2

Hypertension

Anticipatory anxiety best describes the emotion I felt as I arrived at 7:00 a.m. with my fellow medical interns on the first day of my cardiology residency. After orientation, an administrator shepherded us to the hospital floor to begin our first rotation. Graduating interns happily informed us they had completed all patient management issues and written all the notes, and we would only be responsible for any new consults until the 5:00 p.m. shift change occurred. I was delighted at the news because one of my close friends was getting married that day, and I was anxious to get to the wedding reception. Sadly, this was not be, as we received a new consult at 4:30 p.m. that kept us occupied by our obsessive-compulsive resident until late into the evening.

Our new patient arrived from the emergency room diagnosed with "uncontrolled hypertension." She would become my first management encounter with this prevalent but often challenging disease. An older woman, she anxiously watched me as I entered her hospital room. Remarkably, she was completely free of symptoms, and she was confused and worried because her doctor had insisted that she immediately go to the emergency room from his office because of her elevated blood pressure readings. During my interview, she admitted to poor dietary habits and noncompliance with her medications because they made her feel sick. In addition, she was significantly overweight and had laboratory evidence of diabetes and kidney disease.

We began standard oral medications expecting that she would respond. If successful, I could be on my merry way. Despite additional dosing, we were surprised when her elevated blood pressure would not budge, and our supervising resident's constant orders and handwringing did nothing to alleviate the anxiety in the room. We eventually started intravenous treatment to lower her readings, which gradually improved, and we finally left the hospital after 11:00 p.m., exhausted and frustrated that one patient had caused such consternation and challenge. I had missed the wedding reception, so I decided to research and learn as much as possible about our patient's befuddling disease when I arrived home. I read into the early morning hours in preparation for my next hypertensive patient. In retrospect, I am incredibly grateful that my evening was disrupted. I learned some valuable lessons despite the blow to my social life. Hypertension would become the most frequent illness I would treat throughout my medical career.

Hypertension, or consistently elevated blood pressure measurements, over days or weeks is a prevalent disease throughout the world. It affects nearly one-third of the population in the United States and Great Britain. Remarkably, almost half of all hypertensive individuals remain undiagnosed or ineffectively treated. As a result, it significantly contributes to morbidity and mortality, dramatically impacting overall health in the general population. The World Health Organization has estimated that it contributes to the deaths of over nine million people each year. Although more common in older individuals, hypertension is now being increasingly identified in younger adults and children.

The criteria for the diagnosis of hypertension have changed over the last several years. The latest guidelines from the American

Heart Association suggest that elevated blood pressure is firmly diagnosed at a reading of 140/90 or above, but prehypertension is identified at a level above 120/80. Because of these new criteria from 2017, over 40 percent of the US population is now classified as having hypertension. This statistic is an alarming finding and needs greater scrutiny and analysis. I must admit, however, that I remain quite cynical regarding the pharmaceutical industry's involvement in attempting to influence criteria that involve an increase in the use of their product. Profit motivation should never be part of good-quality healthcare.

It should not be surprising that the incidence of hypertension appears to be strongly linked to the increasing trend in obesity. We know that hypertension is an inflammatory disease, and that decreasing inflammation will frequently positively influence an individual's blood pressure management. Obesity is related to excess fat accumulation. Fat cells release inflammatory factors that lead to inflammation in the body. A beneficial hormone called adiponectin is normally released from the fat cells and reduces the risk of diabetes and other metabolic disorders such as hypertension. It also may have some anti-inflammatory effects in normal concentrations in the body. This hormone is reduced in obesity and lower levels are linked to the development of CAD.

Hypertension is one of the top five reasons for outpatient physician visits in many countries. Consequently, physicians have become adept at recognizing and treating this prevalent medical issue. What may be surprising, however, is the number of treated patients who do not achieve optimum blood pressure control. In 2018, the American Medical Association analyzed data from the National Health and Nutrition Examination Survey conducted between 1999 and 2014 in the United States. Results showed only about 54 percent of adults with hypertension had their blood pressure under control. This means that approximately 46 percent of hypertensive individuals were not adequately treated or did not reach their target blood pressure.

What may be even more surprising, however, is that most physicians utilize only a small number of medications to manage this disease process. I suspect that the primary reason for this phenomenon is that most physicians are familiar with their dosage and side effects. As a cardiologist, I am frequently consulted for more resistant cases of hypertension. I am constantly surprised at how infrequently lifestyle modification has been discussed with these patients by their previous providers. In addition, I frequently see patients on three or four antihypertensive drugs at either insufficient dosage or with conflicting medication interactions.

Many patients have significant side effects related to these medications, which makes it difficult for them to take them as directed. It should not surprise patients or physicians that one of the most common causes of medication failure and inadequate hypertension control is the patient's inability to tolerate or afford antihypertensive medicines. In addition, many prescribed antihypertensive medications require multiple daily schedules for compliance; this is not realistic for many people. Many physicians become very frustrated because of noncompliance issues, and they become autocratic and somewhat demanding when patients raise problems of side effects and affordability. I see this not as a frustration, but as an opportunity for interjecting lifestyle options and the addition of certain foods and supplements as an alternative treatment path. Almost universally, I find patients willing to embrace this treatment pathway, and I am surprised that more physicians have not adopted this approach.

Causes of Hypertension

Hypertension is classified as either primary or secondary. Primary, or "essential," hypertension is by far more common. This classification tends to make me smile ironically because it implies that an illness is an essential or primary component of the patient's health. Nothing could be further from the truth! Essential hypertension is frequently the consequence of poor nutrition, a sedentary lifestyle, alcohol excess, sleep disorders, and obesity, which means it is reversible. Unfortunately, it is much easier and less challenging for the physician and the patient to prescribe medications and restrict sodium intake rather than implement a healthy dietary regimen and a regular low-level exercise program. I find it particularly frustrating and remarkably sad that a largely controllable and potentially preventable disease is exacting a significant toll on overall population health simply because either physicians or patients are unwilling to pursue lifestyle changes as a treatment method.

Secondary hypertension, or high blood pressure caused by another underlying condition, is uncommon, but assessing each patient with newly diagnosed hypertension is essential to exclude a secondary cause. It is often seen in younger patients and those with abrupt and severe hypertension that is very difficult to control. Other secondary manifestations that can provide clues include weight gain, acne, progressive kidney failure, and electrolyte abnormalities. Adrenal tumors or dysfunction are rare but require careful assessment in such patients and include surveillance studies to exclude pheochromocytoma, primary aldosteronism, and Cushing's disease. Certain medications can also provoke hypertension in certain patients. Steroids, nonsteroidal agents such as ibuprofen, and over-the-counter cold and allergy remedies are some medications implicated in secondary hypertension.

Sleep issues also contribute to secondary hypertension. During my career, I have seen a dramatic increase in sleep-related illnesses, particularly obstructive sleep apnea. Sleep deprivation and poor sleep habits have become prevalent causes of secondary hypertension, and sleep apnea can lead to obesity. Thus, screening for sleep apnea and effective treatment can frequently improve hypertension in many patients. Weight loss can also have a dramatic positive influence on these patients. CPAP therapy can be challenging to implement, but I am amazed that patients are more willing to use a CPAP than focus on weight loss, even though it would greatly benefit their sleep apnea.

Regular use of CPAP therapy may help with weight loss and usually reduces, to some extent, the risk of further weight gain. The danger of untreated or undiagnosed sleep apnea cannot be understated. It increases a patient's risk for multiple cardiovascular issues, including an increased risk of death from a cardiovascular event. Therefore, I tend to be diligent in trying to screen and aggressively treat this reversible condition. Patients with obstructive sleep apnea typically have insulin resistance and a much higher risk for diabetes. Adding hypertension to the equation can result in a toxic combination that greatly diminishes the benefit that an elixir can cure.

Some data suggest that some patients may have a genetic predisposition to hypertension. I have never performed any genetic testing as part of the management of these patients. Caffeine has also been attributed to causing hypertension. I am less convinced that caffeine consumption contributes to hypertension, but a simple trial of reduced consumption or short-term abstinence should provide enough information to exclude caffeine as a factor.

So, while caffeine doesn't affect hypertension as much as we think, alcohol is a contributing factor. While wine can lessen anxiety and emotional stress for some individuals, a frequent cause of poorly controlled or resistant hypertension is alcohol use (not to mention other harmful side effects of excessive drinking). I almost always query my patients about alcohol consumption when hypertension is one of the health issues that they face. I have no issue with small to modest consumption of alcohol, and some indirect evidence suggests that alcohol may have a mitigating effect on overall cardiovascular illness. But I remain very cautious in recommending alcohol as a therapeutic tool.

Many patients have the misconception that alcohol is valuable to overall long-term health. I remain very skeptical of its benefits, and I am also acutely aware of the potential abuse of this agent. I rarely demand complete abstinence from alcohol while a patient is on blood pressure medications, but I do emphasize the potential detrimental short- and long-term effects on physical and mental health. I also have learned from extensive experience that patients frequently underestimate their alcohol consumption and food intake. Therefore, I try to set guidelines regarding alcohol use. Generally, no more than 7–10 alcoholic beverages per week for men and 3–7 alcoholic beverages for women are helpful guideposts. It is also much better to space alcohol consumption over the entire week rather than resort to binge drinking. It is also quite reasonable and healthy to avoid alcohol use altogether. But it may be surprising (and somewhat disappointing!) that alcohol abstinence has not been associated with adverse medical outcomes.

Types of Antihypertensives

Many medications treat hypertension, including beta-blockers, ACE inhibitors, angiotensin-receptor blockers, calcium channel blockers, centrally acting agents, alpha-receptor blockers, and diuretics. Remarkably, very few new classes of antihypertensive agents have become available, which may be one reason physicians now feel more comfortable utilizing a small number of agents.

I realize that some readers may skip this section or find it too tedious to understand, but I firmly believe in the power of information. If I am going to start a patient on a long-term medicine, I want everyone to understand the mechanism of action, the likely efficacy for them, and the side effects. High blood pressure is a significant cause of death and cardiovascular illness. I must engage in shared decision-making with my patients. This approach will almost always lead to better medication compliance and improved treatment efficacy.

Beta-blockers are stalwart agents in controlling hypertension for many types of patients. They are frequently used in the presence of underlying CAD or congestive heart failure because they also benefit those conditions. As with everything, beta-blockers have many side effects, including fatigue, erectile dysfunction, and hair loss. Provocation or worsening of asthma or underlying lung disease are also commonly attributed to beta-blockers, but in my experience, this is rare. While they can be beneficial, they are not for everyone. Beta-blockers are typically helpful in younger patients and in those individuals with an increased adrenaline output that is manifested by elevated heart rate and increased cardiac output. Elderly patients, however, may often have underlying degenerative electrical pathway problems with the aging heart, so caution must be utilized when increasing the dosage of beta-blockers in this patient population. Beta-blockers do make it more difficult for the heart to adjust its rate in response to increased activity, which can significantly alter exercise tolerance, especially in active and athletic individuals. Consequently, I am very hesitant to prescribe beta-blocker therapy for active individuals who want to continue with high-level exercise training.

ACE inhibitors primarily work by preventing the production of angiotensin II, a substance that constricts the body's blood vessels and is a significant contributing factor in the development of hypertension for many patients. ACE inhibitors are an excellent choice for modest hypertension and those individuals with diabetes. In my experience, ACE inhibitors are well tolerated, but there is a small but significant incidence of angioedema. This potentially life-threatening side effect can cause tongue and lip swelling and possible airway obstruction. Fortunately, this side effect is rare. More common, however, is the development of a nonproductive cough that worsens at night. Coughing can be a particularly bothersome side effect because it usually keeps the patient and their spouse awake at night. As discussed, this sleep deprivation can make hypertension worse. Other side effects include skin rash, worsening kidney function (in patients with preexisting kidney disease), and elevated potassium levels (especially in diabetic patients). Patients with these conditions must continue periodic monitoring for the long term.

Angiotensin-receptor blockers are prevalent first-line blood pressure medications that are well tolerated and effective for mild hypertension. These agents block the development of the potent arterial constricting hormone angiotensin II on the arterial smooth muscle. They may also block the hormone aldosterone and indirectly have a diuretic effect. In my experience, the antihypertensive effect of these medications is mild to moderate at best. Still, they are good initial agents for patients with mild blood pressure elevations and poor compliance issues. They may cause mild kidney issues or elevated potassium levels in some patients, but the risk of angioedema and cough is much lower.

Calcium channel blockers work by interfering with the flow of calcium in and out of cells. This lowers blood pressure by promoting arterial relaxation or reducing heart rate and muscle contraction. Side effects of these agents include slow heart rate and congestive heart failure. Enhancement of blood pressure reduction can be achieved with magnesium supplementation. Magnesium supplements are good blood pressure agents, and this combination with calcium channel blockers can have an additive effect. I frequently use these medications for moderate hypertension. They are excellent for cardiac patients with symptomatic CAD and heart rhythm problems such as atrial fibrillation.

Centrally acting agents block the outpouring of catecholamines from brain stimulation. Catecholamines are neurohormones such as adrenaline that come from the brain and the adrenals and cause the arteries to constrict. Adrenaline also causes the heart rate to increase, and many of these medications slow the heartbeat. As a result, sedation is common, but this "calming effect" is not always well tolerated. These drugs are excellent add-on therapy, but patients must be warned of the potential brain fog. I generally use them for resistant hypertension, and my initial approach is to use it at bedtime only to test its effectiveness. I explain the benefit of sedation and blood pressure control very positively, so my patients accept this agent in a clear light. Since this has the advantage of offsetting the typical early-morning surge in blood pressure and improving nighttime sleep, it is a pragmatic and scientific approach to treating hypertension. If only it would always work!

    Alpha-receptor blockers work by blocking the alpha-1 adrenergic receptors, leading to the relaxation of smooth muscle cells in blood vessels and other tissues. By doing so, they promote vasodilation and reduce the resistance to blood flow, helping to lower blood pressure and alleviate urinary symptoms associated with benign prostatic hyperplasia (BPH). It's important to note that alpha-blockers can have side effects, such as dizziness, lightheadedness, and low blood pressure, but they do have the added benefit of reducing prostate-related issues in men. Prazosin and doxazocin are the most common and effective agents, which have also been successfully used in patients with post-traumatic stress disorder (PTSD). There is also preliminary experimental evidence that doxazocin may have a cellular effect on age reversal. In my approach, alpha-receptor blockers are an excellent example of targeted treatment of high blood pressure for select patients. Older men with prostate issues and patients with associated PTSD may be good candidates for these agents.

    Diuretics are my least favorite antihypertensive, so I have saved them for last. Diuretics are often one of the most prescribed pills by primary care doctors in their quest to slay the blood pressure dragon. They diminish the absorption of water in the kidneys and create a relative state of dehydration in the body, ostensibly to help the kidneys rid the body of more water, sodium, and potassium so less fluid is in the veins. This effect appears to sound logical. Unfortunately, the net effect on blood pressure is tiny unless very high doses of this medication are utilized. Furthermore, the side effects can be significant in many patients. Muscle cramping and weakness are common. Palpitations and heart rhythm disturbances can develop and can occasionally be life-threatening. Low serum sodium levels are seen more frequently in elderly individuals, and blood sugar elevation can be problematic in some patients. Dehydration is a big concern in my older patients. Diuretics can also result in a significant drop in blood pressure when a patient stands, which can result in falls in the elderly. This is one of my most frequent drugs to strike from a patient's medication list. I realize that I may have many physician detractors who are just waiting to argue away my logic but consider this for a moment: Diuretics deplete two factors (potassium and magnesium) that are integral for healthy blood pressure control. Nutrient diets high in magnesium and potassium are well-known to lower blood pressure. Why give a drug that counteracts this effect? Why prescribe an agent that could cause muscle cramps and prevent a patient from experiencing the therapeutic benefit of exercise? Why provoke blood sugar elevation in some patients? Why run the risk of causing orthostatic hypotension and falls in frail elderly patients? In view of the limited benefits and the frequent side effects, I no longer use these agents and I advise the elderly to steer clear. Leg swelling has many causes and diuretics are frequently not the answer.

As a note, the time of day that blood pressure medications are taken may impact the occurrence of cardiovascular events. The Hygia Chronotherapy trial published in the *European Heart Journal* showed a significant decrease in major cardiac events when patients took at least one of their blood pressure medications at bedtime. I've frequently recommended this option to my patients over the years because of the sedating effects of some common blood pressure medications. It is nice to know that it may have a positive impact on survival and benefit their daily acts of living. It makes sense that cardiac events would be diminished given the circadian rise in blood pressure in most individuals' very early morning hours.

Integrative Approach to Blood Pressure Control

While I consider myself a medication minimalist in blood pressure management for my patients, that does not mean that I accept less-than-ideal values for blood pressure control. Optimizing blood pressure reduces strokes, heart attacks, and premature death. My approach is to optimize the dosage of blood pressure medications, eliminate those medicines that are ineffective or have similar therapeutic effects, and stop medications that are poorly tolerated. Many patients can decrease or eliminate medications when they incorporate specific lifestyle changes into their daily routine. Simple things like improving sleep or reducing stress can substantially improve blood pressure and eliminate the need for medication.

It seems logical that lifestyle changes such as weight loss, regular exercise, and good sleep contribute to reasonable blood pressure control. But even still, I am amazed by the magnitude of these nonpharmacologic actions on blood pressure reduction. Weight loss is almost always associated with significant blood pressure improvement in hypertensive patients. Regular exercise and good sleep can also have a profoundly beneficial effect. Sleep apnea is a frequent cause of "resistant" hypertension, and adequate sleep management often allows me to reduce or eliminate medications for patients who suffer from it.

I often hear patients complain that they cannot lose weight because they cannot exercise. My standard response is that up to 80 percent of blood pressure improvement in obese patients is related to calorie restriction, not exercise. Exercise can be highly beneficial, but patients need to understand that regular exercise does not predict successful weight loss. This fact is seen in studies of overweight marathon runners who generally have minimal or no significant weight changes in the months before or following a marathon.

Please attend an upcoming long-distance running race if you doubt this assertion. You will be amazed at the various sizes and shapes of the participants. Completing a marathon is remarkable, but it does not always correlate with weight loss.

Dietary changes can positively impact blood pressure even if they don't lead to weight loss. The hormone insulin is released in response to sugar intake. One of the effects of high-circulating insulin (as seen in insulin-resistant patients) is that too much sodium is retained in the kidney. This can lead to salt retention, edema, and blood pressure elevation. Low total carbohydrate intake reduces circulating insulin levels in all patients. The diminished influence of insulin on the kidney allows for increased clearance of sodium in the urine. This results in a lowering of blood pressure that is independent of weight loss.

Diets that increase the intake of magnesium and potassium can also be very beneficial. Still, patients with poor kidney function need to be careful with excess potassium intake—as always, clarify dietary information and changes with your primary care medical team. I often recommend avocado and Brazil nuts for their high magnesium content. They also contain very healthy fats. Increasing your vegetables and raw fruit intake is also very beneficial. Arterial inflammation can lead to artery constriction and secondary hypertension. The antioxidants in these healthy foods often reduce inflammation and diminish arterial constriction in the long term.

A few supplements that I use to optimize blood pressure control include CoQ10, vitamin C, aged garlic extract, grape seed extract, and fish oil capsules.

Polyunsaturated fatty acids such as fatty fish, olive oil, and eggs can reduce vascular constriction and improve blood pressure readings.

Anthocyanins, the purple, blue, and red pigments that appear in many vegetables and fruits, also help blood pressure. Some familiar sources of these agents include blueberries, cherries, and pomegranates. It is less clear if elderberry or acai products have benefits for hypertension because research is lacking, but they do contain anthocyanins.

A diet low in fruits may be an independent risk for the development of cardiovascular disease. This hazard is likely related to fruit's known beneficial effects on inflammation. Some of the most valuable fruit varieties include blueberries, pomegranates, apples, grapes, and avocados. These products all contain polyphenols. In addition, clinical evidence suggests that a diet that includes raw fruit may decrease diabetes risk. This is because fruit contains fructose, a type of natural sugar that does not require insulin for metabolism, thus avoiding the spike in insulin caused by foods that are high in refined sugars. High consumption of fruit, however, may have a negative impact on the liver. Fructose does not stimulate insulin release or leptin release. Leptin is a hormone secreted by the fat cells that tells the brain to stop eating (satiety hormone). As you can imagine, people can consume large amounts of fruit without a sense of satiety (think of grapes as an example). This increased consumption can lead to excess calories. Fructose is broken down in the liver and can cause some liver issues, but only in very high amounts. Moderation is very important. On the other hand, fruit is a much better choice than processed or simple sugars. Fructose is also present in high fructose corn syrup and is very harmful to us if this ingredient is consumed long term. Many processed foods have high amounts of high fructose corn syrup.

Not only does raw fruit benefit cardiovascular disease risk, but a study of Swedish women and men also revealed that approximately three daily servings of natural fruit reduced the absolute risk of stroke by 13 percent compared to controls. Multiple studies have also revealed that higher fruit consumption reduces the risk of hypertension and hypertensive incidents.

Hypertension is a prevalent and dangerous long-term medical issue that requires early identification and effective treatment. Fortunately, this diagnosis can be very effectively managed with minimal or no medications in most people if lifestyle and nutritional changes can be made. The beneficial impact of these changes can also significantly alter the trajectory of other medical issues, such as diabetes, dementia, and CAD. Simple management strategies and good food can make for a delightful and palatable approach to this prevalent disease.

Takeaways

1. Hypertension is a common medical issue that is increasing in frequency. Approximately 40 percent of the US population meets this diagnosis's criteria.
2. Lifestyle is a significant factor in the development of hypertension, including poor nutrition, inactivity, weight gain, and sleep disorders.
3. Primary, or "essential," hypertension is the most common type, but searching for secondary causes of this problem is imperative and can be curative in some cases.
4. Targeted supplements offer some opportunity for non-medicine control of blood pressure elevation, but these results are generally modest.
5. Ineffective optimization of blood pressure control can significantly decrease health and survival.
6. Lifestyle modifications can dramatically improve blood pressure control, especially sleep optimization.
7. Dietary adjustments can benefit blood pressure control, especially the targeted addition of fruits and foods containing magnesium.

Chapter 3

Diabetes

Should Cardiologists Treat Diabetes?

Cardiologists are not necessarily recognized as predatory subspecialists. When I began medical school in 1975, the field of cardiology primarily dealt with CAD and its complications. We were the first line of support for patients who suffered heart attacks or required coronary angiography before coronary bypass surgery. Unfortunately, we focused on the endpoint of patients' risk factors when, perhaps, we should have focused on the treatment options that led to obstructive artery narrowing in the first place. We were also at the forefront of heart rhythm abnormalities and congestive heart failure treatment. Still, our scope of practice remained limited to the endpoint of a multidimensional disease process.

Back then, endocrinologists monitored and treated lipid and blood sugar abnormalities. The nephrologists were the hypertension experts. Cardiovascular surgeons treated severe CAD with bypass surgery, replaced defective heart valves, closed holes in the heart, and placed heart pacemakers. The vascular surgeons claimed ownership of all other diseases within the vascular tree.

If nothing else, we cardiologists are a curious and somewhat aggressive lot. The growth of the skill set within the cardiology community has been nothing less than remarkable over the past forty years. While other specialties have primarily remained within their medical "silos," we have taken over the management of lipids, hypertension, vascular and coronary revascularization procedures, and some valvular and other structural abnormalities of the heart. With the advent of angioplasty and coronary stent placement, the treatment of CAD changed dramatically. The natural extension of this procedure extended to the vascular tree. Perhaps to the chagrin of our vascular and cardiac surgeons, cardiologists are now the foremost purveyors of stent placement in the carotid and peripheral arteries. We now replace heart valves and close holes in the heart using catheters placed through small incisions in the groin. We fix aortic aneurysms with stent grafts.

The cardiac electrophysiologist ablates dangerous and common rhythm abnormalities previously controlled only with medications or surgery. Pacemakers are now almost exclusively placed by cardiologists. New devices (leadless pacemakers) are placed directly through the groin into the heart without incisions or pacemaker bulges under the collarbone.

Why do I stray from the topic of this chapter to engage in a history lesson? It is to point out the one glaring area that cardiologists have been hesitant to embrace: the treatment of diabetes. If there is one early marker that can predict poor long-term cardiovascular health, it is insulin resistance. Yet only a tiny minority of cardiologists focus on this diagnosis and its treatment, even though it is the root of so much cardiovascular disease. Part of this hesitancy is related to the vast amounts of time some insulin-requiring diabetics require for management. This skill intimidates most cardiologists because they would need more management exposure and skills. For some, other problems are more important to tackle and treat—we are already stretched thin dealing with all the other areas we appropriated from different specialties. As a result, we seem resigned to allowing others to manage this disease. Sadly, however, overall management of diabetes remains woefully inadequate for most patients and only adds to the burden of diseases. Diabetes is often the first domino to fall and leads to an ongoing cascade of subsequent health issues that are consequences of inflammation.

We remain a specialty that deals primarily in the product of inflammatory disease while being blind to its root cause. We have been immensely successful in extending life and saving lives, profiting greatly from this approach. It is time to embrace the treatment of this one remaining pillar of cardiovascular disease and find innovative ways to convince patients of the value of lifestyle changes and control of insulin resistance. We remain a curious and noble specialty and owe our patients a solution to a disease we largely ignore. We need to overcome our ambivalence and fear and get to work!

The Numbers

When I finished my cardiology training in 1983, 2.5 percent of Americans had been diagnosed with diabetes. The current incidence is 10 percent, which is a staggering fourfold increase in less than forty years.

There are two accepted types of diabetes. Type 1 diabetes is much less common, generally occurs earlier in life, and is thought to have an autoimmune basis. Type I diabetics have a much higher need for insulin because the beta cells that secrete insulin in the pancreas have been destroyed by the immune process. Genetics and viruses may also play a role. Unlike type 2, type 1 is generally not reversible.

Type 2 diabetes is usually acquired over years and is linked to insulin resistance. Lifestyle factors that enhance risk include physical inactivity, obesity, and increased sugar intake. Type 2 diabetes tends to occur later in life and can be associated with high insulin levels due to insulin resistance. Type 2 diabetes can be reversed or controlled without medication if weight loss and lifestyle adjustments are undertaken.

The three most frequent risk factors for type 2 diabetes include obesity, physical inactivity, and cigarette use. Associated medical conditions prominent in diabetic patients include hypertension (68 percent) and high cholesterol (44 percent).

The rate of new diabetes cases and the incidence of prediabetes and insulin resistance continue to rise with no apparent trajectory change in sight. This finding is very concerning because, across all age spectrums, the average years of life lost to diabetes is 4.4. Tragically, the average lifespan is reduced by nearly nine years for those younger than age forty-five. This lifespan reduction may be even more significant in those young individuals less than eighteen years of age. Their incidence of type 2 diabetes has nearly doubled in the last several years, while type I diabetes trends have remained flat in this age group. The message worth shouting is that type 2 diabetes is mainly preventable in children. Parents must know that simple lifestyle and dietary changes could positively impact children's health and academic performance in the long term by reducing the risk of childhood diabetes.

Those at risk remain the more vulnerable individuals who have less access to quality healthcare and healthy food, predominantly minority populations. African Americans and Hispanics are at higher risk for type 2 diabetes, and the Native Indian population is at very high risk. Current cigarette use, obesity, and sedentary lifestyle are more commonly identified in minority populations and are strongly linked to diabetes and insulin resistance. Unfortunately, diabetes incidence is inversely related to a person's level of completed education. Genetics probably plays a small role in the Hispanic population, but most of the causes are related to economic and educational barriers and the lack of healthy food and available exercise sources.

Children in low-income families are at particular risk for early-onset type 2 diabetes and face enormous long-term consequences without early detection and treatment. Food deserts (areas with little access to healthy and affordable food options) and a lack of recreational exercise spaces contribute to this risk. Childhood obesity is higher among minority populations, predominantly Hispanic and African American children, and is variously linked to genetic, epigenetic, behavioral, and economic factors. However, it is encouraging to note that education programs can significantly benefit this high-risk group. Healthcare dollars are well spent on educational initiatives for high-risk groups, and the long-term benefits both to individuals and to the financial status of the Medicare program can be enormous.

The economic burden of diabetes currently consumes one in every four healthcare dollars in the United States, and it is likely to increase over the next twenty years. The most significant cost burden is for diabetic patients over sixty-five. Our Medicare system will not be sustainable if this cost continues to rise. Overall, healthcare dollars spent by people with diabetes is on average 2.3 times more than nondiabetics, which is particularly onerous for older retired diabetics on fixed incomes. Many of my older diabetic patients lament that their "golden years" are spent in physicians' offices and at the pharmacy waiting in lines. Despite these lamentations, they often remain unwilling to incorporate lifestyle adjustments that could alleviate their health costs. I remain perplexed and frustrated at this dynamic. This disease was one of my motivations to write this book as an information source to help to make patients' golden years truly enriched and happy.

The incidence and cost of diabetes is alarming enough, then on top of that, diabetes is the primary cause of chronic kidney disease, and approximately 33 percent of people with diabetes have evidence of this problem. Dialysis is a long-term consequence for some patients. African Americans are especially vulnerable to this complication—35 percent of all dialysis patients are African Americans, even though they constitute only 13 percent of the population. It appears that chronic kidney disease may independently worsen the magnitude of diabetes, perhaps because of elevated blood urea nitrogen in the bloodstream, which may enhance insulin resistance.

If the healthcare profession is to have any impact on the devastating consequences of diabetes, we must identify and aggressively treat the root causes. As a cardiologist, I freely admit that I was blind to the importance of prevention because I was excited to treat the acute consequences of this disease. It was as if I was the eager young firefighter who reveled in the treatment of a house fire, only later to recognize the devastation of the loss to the homeowner. Preventing the hazards of a medical "home fire" was not on my radar early on in my career, and I now need to make up lost ground and help all patients avoid future tragedies. We must change the paradigm if we are to have any impact on the well-being of our patients. This change of direction is a struggle for the masses of cardiovascular specialists with a reactionary philosophy. Yet we must heed the wisdom of Henry David Thoreau: "There are a thousand hacking at the branches of evil to one who is one striking at the root."

Insulin Resistance

Insulin resistance affects nearly 50 percent of the adult population in the United States. That is a staggering number considering the consequences of these abnormalities. The likelihood that an individual with insulin resistance will eventually develop diabetes is very high unless proactive measures are undertaken. The good news is that insulin resistance is mainly treatable with lifestyle changes. The bad news is that insulin resistance is *primarily* treatable with lifestyle changes!

The basic premise regarding insulin resistance is that the passive movement of glucose into the cells is impaired due to a problem with the inner cell glucose transport.

Essentially, insulin resistance is like the effects of inflation on the economy. Insulin's overall "purchasing power" to move sugar (goods and services) into the cells is decreased. The consequence of this reduced effectiveness of insulin leads to an overabundance of circulating glucose (goods) unless there is an increase in insulin (increased money supply) to overcome the imbalance. The problem is that the surplus of insulin has only limited benefits if the supply of sugar (goods) continues to flood the body through poor eating habits and gluconeogenesis in the liver. Persistent blood sugar elevation eventually causes pathologic changes in our vascular system, brain, and liver, many of which are potentially irreversible. Just as inflation can cause eventual economic collapse, insulin resistance can eventually lead to multi-organ inflammation and potentially catastrophic events such as heart attacks and strokes. Applying disciplinary measures to curb these excesses is the only way to overcome the disease burden.

Insulin resistance is when the body's cells don't respond well to insulin, which helps regulate blood sugar levels. It's a critical factor in conditions like type 2 diabetes.

There are two main types of insulin resistance: one that affects the liver (hepatic) and one that affects skeletal muscles.

Hepatic insulin resistance means that the liver doesn't respond appropriately to insulin's instructions. Usually, insulin tells the liver to stop producing glucose (sugar), but when the liver becomes resistant to insulin, it continues making too much glucose. This leads to high blood sugar levels, which is a problem in diabetes.

Skeletal muscle insulin resistance means the muscles don't efficiently take in glucose from the blood, even when insulin is present. This flaw appears to be related to the impairment of the activation and migration process that results in the passive movement of sugar into the cells and subsequent consolidation into glycogen. This also contributes to high blood sugar levels.

While both types of insulin resistance are important, hepatic insulin resistance is considered more critical. The liver has a significant role in regulating blood sugar levels, and when it doesn't respond well to insulin, it produces too much glucose, causing further problems.

It's important to understand that both types of insulin resistance can affect each other and contribute to metabolic issues. So, to fully grasp insulin resistance, it's necessary to consider both the liver and skeletal muscle aspects.

The newest proposition regarding impaired glucose transport inside the cell appears related to the breakdown of circulating triglycerides to diacylglycerol. This compound partially blocks the receptor cascade mechanism that allows glucose absorption inside the cell.

Elevated triglycerides appear to occur because of insulin's impact on converting ingested carbohydrates into fatty acids. This process is called de novo lipogenesis (DNL). These available fatty acids are joined together into circulating fats in the plasma called triglycerides. High circulating insulin levels can convert the excess carbohydrates from a high-sugar meal into triglycerides. High liver insulin and peripheral insulin resistance also reduce HDL (good cholesterol) production and circulating levels, increasing the risk of atherosclerotic vascular disease. I frequently use the triglyceride/HDL ratio to assess patient risk for future cardiac events. A ratio of greater than two is associated with an increased risk threshold. A higher ratio is also a good tool for predicting insulin resistance.

The increased circulating glucose that cannot pass directly into the skeletal muscle for glycogen storage is distributed to the liver and converted to fat. The chronic result of this process is nonalcoholic fatty liver disease (the most common cause of underlying liver disease). Unfortunately, there appears to be a link between this chronic liver inflammation and the subsequent development of end-stage liver disease and possibly liver cancer.

Insulin's effect on glucose metabolism primarily involves three cellular systems. These three primary affected cells are the skeletal muscle, fat, and liver cells. Insulin helps sugar (glucose) enter our body's cells. The cells mainly affected by insulin for sugar transport are muscle cells and fat cells. In muscle cells, insulin acts like a key that unlocks the doors of the cells to allow glucose inside. The muscles use this glucose for energy and other essential functions. Similarly, insulin in fat cells helps open the doors to let glucose in. The glucose is then stored in the fat cells as an energy reserve. These muscle and fat cells are the primary places where insulin works to transport sugar.

Insulin has two main effects on the liver:

1. Tells the liver to reduce the production of glucose (sugar): When insulin levels are normal and working correctly, it signals the liver to slow down or stop making glucose. This helps keep the blood sugar levels in balance.
2. Promotes the storage of excess glucose as glycogen: When there's extra glucose in the bloodstream, insulin helps the liver store it as glycogen. Think of glycogen as a storage form of glucose. Later, when the body needs energy, the liver can break down glycogen and release glucose into the bloodstream. In simple terms, insulin tells the liver to stop making too much glucose and helps store the extra glucose as a backup energy source. This way, insulin helps maintain a stable blood sugar level.

When we have excess glucose (sugar) in our body, it can be stored in two different ways in the liver:

1. Glycogen storage: This is like a temporary energy bank. When we have extra glucose, the liver takes it and stores it as glycogen. Later, when our body needs quick energy, the liver can break down the glycogen and release glucose into the bloodstream.
2. Making fat: If more glucose can be stored as glycogen, the liver can convert the excess glucose into fat. This fat is then stored in fat cells throughout the body, acting as a long-term energy reserve.

A fatty liver is a condition with too much fat in the liver cells. One of the processes that can contribute to fat accumulation in the liver is DNL, as mentioned above. Think of DNL as a process where the liver produces new fat from excess sugars (carbohydrates) in our body. When we consume more sugars than our body needs for energy, the liver can convert the extra sugars into fat. This fat gets stored in the liver cells, leading to fatty liver. In conditions like nonalcoholic fatty liver disease (NAFLD), which is commonly associated with obesity and metabolic problems, the liver can have a higher rate of DNL. This means the liver produces more fat than usual, which adds to the fatty liver condition. DNL is just one piece of the puzzle regarding fatty liver, and other factors are involved. Things like unhealthy diet, inflammation, and genetics can also contribute to fatty liver.

To manage fatty liver, lifestyle changes are often recommended. This may include making healthier food choices, reducing the intake of excess sugars and fats, losing weight (if needed), and being physically active. By making these changes, we can help reduce the production of new fat in the liver and improve the condition of fatty liver.

It is also essential to understand that two different glucose transporters facilitate the migration of glucose across the lipid cell membrane. These transporters are facilitated diffusion glucose transporters (GLUTs) and sodium-glucose linked transporters (SGLTs). Why is it important to understand these transporters?

Obesity is a complex process. It is essential to recognize that a cascade of many different hormonal and enzymatic processes is engaged in the metabolism of glucose and fat production. I am hopeful that improved knowledge of the entire metabolic process of energy production and preservation will allow patients to understand diet's impact on energy storage.

Imagine blood glucose as a boxcar on a train track. This boxcar is filled with essential energy materials that our bodies need. But it won't serve any purpose if it just travels around the bloodstream without reaching its destination. To get the energy from glucose into our cells, we need unique engines called GLUTs that work in conjunction with circulating insulin levels. These transporters latch on to the boxcars and pull them inside the cells. Once inside, the boxcars are unloaded, and their valuable materials are used for various cellular functions.

Now, let's say the boxcars contain crucial materials that are needed continuously but cannot reach the cell's "station" due to low carbohydrate intake. This low carbohydrate intake results in low insulin levels, so the transporters cannot work effectively. In this situation, the cells need an alternative energy source. This is where DNL comes into play. When carbohydrate intake is low, the body can activate DNL inside the cell, which creates new fat (lipids) from other sources, such as excess dietary protein or stored carbohydrates (glycogen). This fat is an alternative energy reserve for cellular processes when glucose availability is limited.

The fat produced through DNL is stored inside the cells as a cellular adaptive mechanism. It gives the body an alternative energy source when glucose is scarce. This fat can be used later to provide energy for cellular functions. One can see that DNL is an essential process in energy balance during low-carbohydrate states like starvation, but DNL can also be harmful when excess fat is stored during periods of high carbohydrate intake.

These different transporters act like little tools that help move sugar (glucose) into different cells. GLUTs are found in the small intestine, kidneys, skeletal muscles, heart muscle, brain, and fat cells and work in complex ways within these cells to allow a significant increase in the movement of sugar into the cells. Without these vital tools, the movement of glucose into the cells would be limited.

Another essential transporter called SGLT2 is primarily found in our kidneys. Its job is to absorb sugar back into our bloodstream. However, certain medications called SGLT2 inhibitors work by blocking this transporter. By blocking SGLT2, these medications prevent the reabsorption of sugar as it passes through the kidneys, so they have been found to be effective in treating diabetes.

Interestingly, researchers have discovered an additional benefit of these SGLT2 inhibitors. They seem to improve the longevity (long-term health) of patients with congestive heart failure. This is likely because these medications also help reduce insulin resistance, which is a problem in conditions like diabetes. It's possible that these secondary benefits of SGLT2 inhibitors may extend to other patients as well, not just those with congestive heart failure. By reducing insulin resistance, these medications may have positive effects on overall health and longevity.

So, in simple terms, GLUTs are like little tools that help move sugar into cells, and SGLT2 inhibitors are medications that prevent sugar from being reabsorbed in the kidneys. These medications not only help with diabetes but also appear to provide additional benefits, such as improving heart health and potentially extending lifespan, by reducing insulin resistance.

Blood sugar balance involves complex mechanisms that are only now being better understood. What we do understand is that dietary indiscretions can dramatically overload our body's capacity to transport glucose inside the cell for energy utilization.

It is also known that insulin is not significantly influential on the cellular influx of glucose into liver cells. Rather, insulin's primary role is to reduce the production of new glucose. This effect is essential to understand because insulin has a limited role in various biological processes within our body.

The influence of insulin is critical to maintaining sensitive energy balance and energy delivery within the vital organs. It must be seen as one of the many important players in an orchestra constantly performing within our bodies. Any imbalance or depletion of the orchestra members will completely distort the beauty of the music in much the same way that our cellular performance becomes distorted through inflammatory changes.

Advanced Glycation End Products (AGE)

When discussing diabetes and inflammation, it is important to discuss AGEs. AGEs are harmful agents formed when sugar combines with fats or proteins. These damaging molecules can be either produced internally or consumed from external sources.

Internal production of these products occurs when blood sugars are chronically elevated. The overabundance of sugar concentration allows these excess sugars to bind to the bloodstream's circulating fats or amino acids. This initial combination can be reversed if our blood sugar comes down. If blood sugar levels remain high, further chemical reactions occur that make the process irreversible. The resultant AGE molecules bind to receptors on the cell wall called RAGE receptors. This binding process leads to an "angry" reaction within the cell that releases a cascade of pro-inflammatory mediators. If our blood sugar remains high long term, secondary to insulin resistance, this chronic inflammatory activity will advance aging. It is recognized that the production and consumption of AGEs are linked to the development of many inflammatory diseases that include vascular disease, CAD, kidney disease, and possibly Alzheimer's dementia.

We may unknowingly consume high levels of AGEs in our diet, especially in foods cooked at high temperatures (280–330 degrees Fahrenheit). Any method that causes a browning effect on foods—like grilling, searing, frying, and broiling—can produce AGEs. For example, the number of AGEs in one fried egg is almost thirty times greater than in an egg scrambled in olive oil at a low temperature. Why is this so? It has to do with temperature. A high temperature is required to fry an egg, but you typically make scrambled eggs at a lower temperature. High temperature is the key to more AGE production. That is why grilling at high temperatures is bad for us! Bacon has one of the highest numbers of AGE of all prepared foods. One can imagine the potential inflammatory environment inflicted on the early-morning body when bacon and fried eggs are on the menu! Dietary consumption is the most prevalent source of these harmful products, but if patients know about them and their effects, they could reduce their exposure and improve their health and longevity.

Some other foods are high in AGEs, including dairy products (butter and cheese), highly processed foods, products high in saturated fats, and fast foods. It must be clearly understood that food habits that lead to chronic blood sugar elevation may be associated with the development of AGEs internally. Remember that AGEs form in the presence of elevated blood sugar. Chronic ingestion of "healthy" fruits that provoke significant sugar spikes (grapes, bananas, mango) can allow the abnormal proteins to bind to the sugar and offset the beneficial effects of fruit as an alternative to processed foods. So again, it comes down to the concept of moderation and diversity when considering the ideal diet for everyone. My real intention in discussing the role of AGEs in chronic inflammation and disease is to introduce the additional importance of food preparation as everyone transitions to a healthy dietary practice. The ultimate long-term goal is to reduce the risk of insulin resistance and diabetes. Reducing AGE bioavailability in our bodies can go a long way to mitigate disease risk.

Approaches to Reduce AGE Production

Specific B vitamins may inhibit internal AGE formation in certain circumstances. For example, benfotiamine, the synthetic version of thiamine, blocks AGE absorption in the gut. It is still being determined if supplementation with these nutrients has a significant effect. Still, it may be a reasonable option if you are worried about the long-term effects of AGEs. Adding acidic agents such as lemon juice and vinegar in food preparation also reduces the resultant number of generated AGEs. Some limited research also suggests that regular exercise may reduce the bioavailability of circulating AGEs or reduce the secondary consequences of inflammation and arterial damage. Older individuals and those with kidney disease appear to be particularly susceptible to the harmful effects of AGE production. Consumption and lifestyle changes to lessen their impact can be highly advantageous in preserving healthy aging.

Food preparation techniques such as stewing, poaching, steaming, and boiling can significantly reduce AGE generation, as can marinating in an acidic environment (vinegar or lemon juice), cooking at lower temperatures for a shorter duration, and adding certain spices such as turmeric. Some plants contain beneficial antioxidant compounds called polyphenols. Consumption of these plants and fruits that are high in resveratrol (raspberries, grapes, blueberries) combined with supplementing with quercetin and vitamin C can lower the number of absorbed AGEs. Most days of the week, regular exercise reduces AGE levels, especially in older and more susceptible individuals. Together, these relatively simple lifestyle methods can immediately lower the risk of inflammation and significantly decrease the risk of insulin resistance and subsequent diabetes.

Air frying is a popular cooking method these days. This technique produces high temperatures quickly. I don't have any scientific data, but my sense is that it would increase AGE production due to the high temperature that develops during the cooking process.

If you are serious about making a concerted effort to preserve your long-term health, recognize that insulin resistance is your enemy, and these lifestyle changes are part of your defensive strategy. Most individuals would never need my services if they could generate the enthusiasm and perseverance to embrace these methods. Although I am pragmatic and realize that outdoor grilling is an American tradition, I suggest it becomes a special event rather than a standard practice so that everyone can occasionally enjoy the savory flavor of a grilled piece of meat. Adding the marination process can enhance the flavor and lower the risk, so enjoy your occasional reward. You deserve it!

Treatment Options for Diabetes

Unfortunately, many physicians ignore or minimize the root cause of the disorder when talking to a newly diagnosed patient, and the effect (elevated blood sugar) becomes the treatment objective. With that objective in mind, doctors will recommend dietary changes emphasizing calorie restriction and carbohydrate reduction and tell patients to lose weight, exercise, and begin taking medications. They don't fully explain the role of hormones such as insulin, and they don't discuss any more lifestyle changes. Instead, they turn to medication.

The vast number of drugs now available to control diabetes is beyond the scope of this book, but I advise you to educate yourself with the excellent resources that are readily available on various websites. However, I would like to summarize some of the successful drug treatments with different target sites and objectives of therapy because it may help to better understand the evolution of diabetic medicine in the future. I have withheld specific drug names because they are too numerous to list.

Drug therapy today is targeted at three primary objectives: 1) increasing the available insulin, 2) enhancing insulin sensitivity at the cellular level, and 3) decreasing available glucose in the bloodstream. Hormonal manipulation and targeting are the most recent approach to treatment. This medical treatment approach will be the focus of my efforts to help you comprehend this rather complex approach to care.

Standard treatment for newly diagnosed diabetes is often dictated by a persistent fasting blood sugar level or a moderate elevation of the glycohemoglobin (also known as the hemoglobin A1c) blood test. The glycohemoglobin level is a non-fasting test that reflects the average blood sugar level. Any value of 6.5 or greater is indicative of overt diabetes, and values between 5.7 and 6.4 are considered prediabetic values.

When someone is newly diagnosed with diabetes, treatment usually starts with a medication called metformin. Metformin helps cells take in more sugar, and it's generally safe with few side effects. It doesn't cause a significant drop in blood sugar levels and may even lead to weight loss. However, it can increase the risk of vitamin B12 deficiency, which can cause nerve problems. Metformin has also been reported to enhance longevity in some studies, but this benefit remains unclear. It is essential to use metformin only for treating diabetes, as its long-term benefits for nondiabetic purposes are still uncertain.

Other medications used for diabetes include sulfonylureas and meglitinides, which help the pancreas release more insulin. These medications can cause low blood sugar levels and weight gain.

Thiazolidinediones improve insulin sensitivity in cells but can cause weight gain and may affect the heart.

Another group of medications, alpha-glucosidase inhibitors, reduces sugar absorption in the digestive tract. However, they can lead to discomfort and gas.

Certain medications work by enhancing the presence of insulin. These drugs target hormones known as incretins, increasing insulin release, and reducing liver sugar production. Examples of these medications are DPP-4 inhibitors and GLP-1 receptor agonists. They don't cause weight gain and may even promote weight loss.

SGLT2 inhibitors, or gliflozins, are newer medications that lower blood sugar levels by preventing the kidneys from reabsorbing glucose. They can lead to weight loss and may benefit diabetic patients with heart failure. However, they increase the risk of vaginal infections and may slightly increase the risk of amputations in high-risk patients.

Insulin may be necessary to control blood sugar levels if other treatments don't work. Insulin therapy can be challenging, as it requires careful dosing and timing, and it often leads to weight gain, which can worsen the patient's condition.

Some natural means to lower your blood sugar remain relatively safe if you carefully monitor blood sugar levels and you are not pregnant and do not have significant underlying kidney disease. Magnesium is essential to glucose and insulin homeostasis, and low magnesium levels are associated with insulin resistance. Magnesium replacement plays a role in the movement of glucose into the cells and can assist with a lowering of blood sugar levels. Most patients should consider taking 300–400 mg of magnesium daily should be considered in most patients but used cautiously in patients with kidney insufficiency and only under the approval of their healthcare provider.

Cinnamon and zinc are beneficial in lowering blood sugar levels, and zinc has the added benefit of improving immunity. Cinnamon may also lower cholesterol levels. Berberine is an effective plant derivative that can improve insulin resistance and has somewhat similar effects to metformin. It should be used carefully while on prescription drugs and not by children. Apple cider vinegar has many uses, including lowering blood sugar. Gymnema is an exciting plant derivative that has multiple effects on blood sugar, including a decrease in the taste of sugary foods, a reduction in glucose absorption in the gut, and modest stimulation of insulin release by the pancreas. Careful blood sugar monitoring is essential if a diabetic patient begins to explore these options. This can be achieved with fingerstick blood glucose testing or continuous glucose monitoring devices that are now readily available. Consultation with individual healthcare providers is also advised.

When it comes to treating such a prevalent disease as diabetes, an integrative attitude that looks at root causes and aggressively works to thwart the onset and destructive consequences of insulin resistance will go a long way toward gaining control. Still, it will take much education and coaching to get there. I spend significant time educating my patients on lifestyle modifications and the impending consequences of insulin resistance. While I am uncertain if the time is well spent in many cases, I know that physicians must lead the way. The goal is threefold: prevention, prevention, and prevention! This theme is one that motivated me to write this book. If I can explain it logically, I hope patients will understand the long-term benefits, so physicians do not have to treat these chronic and sometimes devastating consequences.

It is an exciting opportunity for physicians to work with patients who are open to making significant lifestyle changes, such as adjusting their diet and committing to regular exercise. While it can be challenging when patients initially struggle to implement these changes, I've seen many newly diagnosed individuals demonstrate a strong desire to succeed. Collaborating with these patients can be a fulfilling experience, as we work together to achieve their health goals. It's important to remember that treatment requires effort and commitment, but the rewards of a healthy and active life are well worth it. By taking the initiative to make positive changes in our lives, we can set ourselves up for a lifetime of good health and happiness. Let's be role models for our loved ones and show them that we're committed to enjoying a vibrant and disease-free future together.

These are not idle wishes. They are attainable goals. Diabetes can be easily controlled and often cured with a strong willingness to eat healthier, exercise, and focus on ideal body weight. Let us all begin!

<u>Takeaways</u>

1. Cardiologists have taken over the treatment of most underlying cardiovascular risk factors, and they need to consider diabetes as their new frontier of management.
2. The incidence of diabetes is exploding, especially among children. This future burden of disease predicts a high incidence of cardiovascular illnesses.
3. One in four healthcare dollars are consumed by direct or indirect treatment of diabetes and insulin resistance.
4. Insulin resistance is the precursor of diabetes and affects nearly 50 percent of the population.
5. AGEs are toxins formed between circulating sugar and food proteins and fats. High-temperature cooking can cause them. Reducing these toxins is vital to lowering cardiovascular risk.
6. Insulin resistance is likely one of the most significant factors in the development of cardiovascular disease. Understanding the role of insulin and the cause of insulin resistance is essential to reduce risk and facilitate treatment.
7. Many drugs target diabetes control. The most effective treatments, however, are lifestyle adjustments that include exercise, reduced sugar intake, and other important lifestyle

modifications.
8. Magnesium, berberine, zinc, and cinnamon are some of the nutrients that may have a complementary role in glucose control.

Chapter 4

Sleep

When I embarked on my medical residency, I knew it would be both an exciting and somewhat intimidating experience. Experienced residents hammered home that I should expect long hours and sleepless nights. Sleep came at a premium as work hours and night calls multiplied. While I was young and felt invincible in many ways, sleep deprivation began to take a heavy toll as the months of nonstop work progressed. Sickness, irritability, emotional outbursts, and anger became commonplace among my intern group.

The pinnacle of my sleep deprivation occurred in the deep winter months as I struggled to survive an incredibly busy three-month heart surgery rotation. We were expected to be available twenty-four hours a day, seven days a week. My hospital day began at 6:30 a.m. and frequently ended close to midnight. I would also take calls throughout the night, disrupting what little sleep I did get. For the last several weeks of the rotation, I was functioning on a nightly sleep allowance of three hours per night with frequent beeper interruptions. I was constantly fatigued and hungry, but I lost weight because I had no time to buy groceries or fix meals. My irritability skyrocketed, and my hygiene and interpersonal relationships suffered greatly. I felt indebted to God's grace for helping me avoid significant medical errors during this period. I experienced firsthand the consequences of sleep loss on health, but I failed to recognize the detrimental impact that it caused on my well-being.

As I conducted research for this book, I was surprised that sleep dysfunction was among the most influential contributors to cardiovascular disease. (I did notice the rather high incidence of sleep apnea signs in many of my patients throughout the years, and this allowed me to recognize the secondary consequences on cardiovascular and overall metabolic health. After much research, I have been screening for sleep apnea for over fifteen years.) This information was particularly important to me personally because of my lifestyle of long days, short nights, and call-related sleep deprivation, which has continued even after residency. The physician is expected to be the purveyor of healing. Still, it is hard for an interventional cardiologist to avoid late-night and early-morning emergencies that require treating a heart attack.

Physicians are not immune to bad habits or the consequences of an erratic lifestyle, including those that affect decision-making skills and interpersonal relationships. A study of sleep-deprived general surgeons revealed that their surgery times were 14 percent longer with a 20 percent increased error rate. Despite this scientific evidence, physicians are not required to follow the same sleep regulations that airline pilots and other transportation workers adhere to. The overall impact of sleep deprivation on medical errors, misaligned interpersonal skills, and depression is likely underestimated. Jesus's words in Luke, Chapter 4 — "Physician, heal thyself"—must remind physicians to practice the art of healing themselves to serve their patients better.

Just like many of the nutritional and exercise benefits that have been discussed so far in this book, good sleep hygiene is vital for everyone as we pursue long-term health. What constitutes my definition of good sleep hygiene?

I teach my patients the importance of quality sleep for optimum health.

You need to:

- get six to nine hours (maximum) of sleep; seven to eight hours is ideal
- ensure a cool and completely dark environment
- not be in front of a TV, computer, or other screen for at least one hour before sleep
- lower the house lights in preparation for sleep
- not allow your children or pets to share a bed with you on an ongoing basis because it is very disruptive to good-quality sleep
- use white noise, such as a fan or other sound device
- avoid eating food or alcohol within an hour before sleep—this lowers your REM and deep-sleep quality
- try to sleep on your side to reduce the risk of snoring and diminish the risk of sleep apnea
- turn off any lights on bedside devices such as alarm clocks and other devices
- limit any daytime naps to twenty to ninety minutes maximum
- try to go to bed and arise at the same time, no matter what the circumstances ("catching up" on your sleep on weekends frequently disrupts your sleep cycle and may make you more fatigued during the day)

How Sleep Affects Health

If you are not convinced of the link between sleep deprivation and adverse health outcomes, consider these facts related to daylight savings time (DST):

- A 2014 study from the University of Michigan revealed a 24 percent increase in heart attacks on the Monday following DST, when we lose an hour of sleep.
- A 2016 neurology study from Finland identified an 8 percent total increase in stroke in the forty-eight hours after DST, with a 20 percent increased incidence in individuals sixty-five and older.
- A 2009 Bureau of Labor Statistics database evaluation identified increased work-related injuries on Mondays after DST. There also appears to be an increase in fatal and nonfatal accidents on the Monday after we "spring forward."

These studies confirm that losing as little as one hour of sleep can lead to significant health-related issues. Imagine the cumulative effect of chronic sleep deprivation on individual health!

Sleep is a somewhat complex process directly related to our circadian rhythm. Humans as a species are meant to sleep when it's dark. The primary sleep hormone, melatonin, is regulated by light exposure and is released as sunlight disappears. Melatonin production and release are also affected by early-morning sun exposure (6:00–8:30 a.m.). Early-morning sunlight exposure (ideally outside) causes an increase in daytime melatonin production that helps us to fall asleep more easily in the evening. Melatonin has many different functions, including anti-inflammatory and antioxidant effects. It induces our brain to prepare for bed, but its anti-inflammatory properties may also protect against cardiac events as we sleep. Sleep studies have revealed a significant rise in at least one pro-inflammatory cardiac marker as sleep deprivation increases.

Multiple hormonal changes occur because of poor sleep habits, including increased cortisol levels, fasting insulin levels, and decreased hormone production. It is important to understand the impact of sleep on overall health. For example, during deep sleep, also known as slow-wave sleep or stage 3 of non-REM sleep, several vital processes occur in the body. The body repairs and regenerates tissues, muscles, and bones. Deep sleep is crucial in immune function, hormone regulation, and memory consolidation. It is associated with the release of growth hormone, which is essential for growth and development and tissue repair. Furthermore, deep sleep is believed to be involved in the maintenance of healthy brain function. It supports cognitive processes such as learning, memory, and problem-solving and is important for emotional well-being and mood regulation.

In terms of physical changes, during deep sleep, the heart rate and breathing slow down, and blood pressure drops. This reduction in physiological activity allows the body to conserve energy and promote rest and recovery.

Overall, deep sleep is a vital stage of the sleep cycle that contributes to overall health and well-being. It is essential for physical restoration, immune function, memory consolidation, and optimal brain function. If the body does not have the chance to repair itself, cellular dysfunction and hormonal imbalance will occur. Numerous studies have revealed a significant increase in various inflammatory markers when sleep deprivation is present. All these inflammatory markers have been linked to detrimental effects on long-term health, including many already discussed in this book. Simply improving sleep hygiene can significantly impact health and longevity.

As has been discussed, inflammation is the primary driver of CAD, and chronic sleep deprivation markedly enhances this risk. Sleep deprivation also provokes insulin resistance, resulting in high blood sugar levels. Elevated cortisol levels and enhanced sympathetic nervous system activity also occur with sleep deprivation. These hormonal changes can lead to significant nocturnal blood pressure elevation. This is one of the reasons why heart attacks and strokes occur most frequently in the early morning hours in patients who are chronically sleep deprived.

Multiple studies have revealed an increased risk of chronic cardiovascular risk factors, such as diabetes, hypertension, and sleep apnea, in individuals who have poor sleep habits. A fourteen-year study of over two thousand Japanese men aged thirty-five to fifty-four revealed a greater than threefold increased risk of cardiovascular events in men who slept less than six hours per night. In addition, a large European study of nearly a half million men and women revealed a 45 percent increased risk of developing or dying of coronary heart disease (CHD) and a 15 percent greater risk of stroke in those individuals who slept for less than five to six hours. Interestingly, there was also a significant risk of stroke and CHD in those individuals who slept more than eight to nine hours. Despite this convincing evidence, sleep is not considered a significant factor in most clinics when assessing patients with underlying cardiovascular disease.

It is also recognized that night shift work is associated with an increased risk of obesity, especially central obesity. This would place night shift workers at higher risk for sleep apnea and its attendant complications. This group of individuals should be a focus of treatment if physicians and employers desire an enhancement in health promotion among their populations.

Quality and Quantity of Good Sleep

Several observational studies have shown a strong link between longevity and sleep duration. There appears to be a U-shaped curve that reveals that the ideal sleep duration is seven to eight hours per night. The Centers for Disease Control has shown that more than 60 percent of US adults sleep less than eight hours per night. The average sleep duration for most Americans is approximately 6.5 hours. Individuals who spend more than nine hours in bed have a shorter lifespan and an increased risk of diabetes. In addition, older women appear to have a lower lifespan when they spend over nine hours in bed. This is probably related to multiple factors and underlying conditions, but the takeaway is that oversleeping in older adults is unhealthy and may even be lethal. For those who do get the suggested seven to eight hours of sleep, any positive effect on longevity assumes that the quality of sleep is high. Unfortunately, time spent in bed does not always equate to good-quality sleep.

It has been recognized for decades that sleep includes several phases. Most sleep experts agree that the first two hours are critically important. Deep sleep generally occurs within thirty to forty minutes of falling asleep, is the most restorative stage, and is associated with the release of human growth hormone. This critically important phase allows for cellular repair and rejuvenation and eliminates the sense of sleepiness that would otherwise occur during waking hours. Sleep before midnight is crucial to our well-being if we all try to follow our body's normal circadian rhythm, because this time-frame is when the human body is programmed to obtain the greatest amount of crucial deep sleep. REM sleep is also essential because this is the stage when our brain stores memories and processes our thoughts and emotions. This "dream phase" is critical for our mood, concentration, and long-term memory retention.

Deep sleep and REM sleep constitute a small portion of total sleep duration and can be measured as a percentage. Higher values are excellent and usually indicate a high-quality sleep pattern.

A decrease in either of these two sleep stages becomes significantly problematic to our immunity and can lead to chronic inflammation and increased risk of infections. Most of us recognize that a weekend of poor sleep related to increased alcohol, late nights, and poor eating habits will often lead to a subsequent viral infection. Our bodies are good teachers, and we must become wise and attentive pupils.

In my practice, I try to focus not only on a patient's sleep duration, but also on the quality of their sleep. Sleep apnea is prevalent and not exclusive to overweight individuals. Undiagnosed or untreated sleep apnea is a significant cause of insulin resistance, inflammation, resistant hypertension, and cardiovascular disease. Since patients themselves might not always be the best judges of the quality of their sleep, it is very beneficial to have a spouse or partner present during my interviews with patients to clarify the presence or absence of sleep-related illness. It is now known that even mild decreases in oxygen saturation during sleep can impact long-term memory, resulting in cognitive dysfunction, and dementia. Nocturnal oxygen screening has been suggested for all patients who may have risk factors for dementia.

REM sleep is critically important in the development of higher-learning capabilities. Research suggests that more than one alcoholic beverage can significantly impact REM duration in many individuals. This becomes particularly important when students or workers have a significant test or presentation on the day following moderate or high alcohol consumption. A large segment of the population chooses to drink alcohol for its relaxing qualities. The impact of moderate alcohol consumption on overall sleep quality has been measured and appears to be adverse. In addition, nightly alcohol use can have a cumulative effect on overall sleep quality and, therefore, on cognition. This doesn't mean that small amounts of alcohol are always harmful to sleep quality. Still, one can imagine the impact of heavy alcohol use during a weekend celebration and subsequent worker performance in the days following this activity. This is particularly true for drivers and students.

Younger and middle-aged men would also be surprised to learn that there is evidence that reduced REM sleep and poor sleep quality induced by alcohol consumption reduce testosterone levels and measurable testicular size. This may impact fertility and the development of excess fat around the abdomen, also known as belly fat.

Sleep deprivation can:

- potentially impact fertility, although the relationship between the two is complex and not fully understood (it's important to note that infertility is a multifaceted issue, and sleep deprivation alone is unlikely to be the sole cause of infertility—other factors such as age, underlying medical conditions, lifestyle factors, and overall health play significant roles in fertility)
- disrupt the body's hormonal balance, including hormones involved in reproductive processes
- affect the production and regulation of reproductive hormones such as testosterone, estrogen, and progesterone
- lead to increased stress levels and decreased immune function, indirectly affecting fertility
- contribute to conditions such as irregular menstrual cycles, ovulatory dysfunction, and increased risk of reproductive disorders

Sleep and Cognitive Function

Some essential caveats can be drawn from the extensive scientific data. There's a strong link between sleep deprivation and cognitive function. Lack of sleep can dramatically affect simple skills such as driving and test-taking. Research indicates that approximately 30 percent of heavy truck accidents appear to be directly related to fatigue. This causation is more significant than drug and alcohol use in this framework. This is critically important information for those individuals who are greatly concerned about developing Alzheimer's disease or other cognitive dysfunctions later in life.

In the past, being able to perform and excel with only minimal sleep was often considered a "red badge of courage." This falsehood may be sustainable for a period, but the long-term consequences can be rather dramatic. Performance science has been leading the way in the benefits of sleep for several years. That is why professional athletes have been strongly encouraged to get significant amounts of sleep during seasons of high-level performance. One can learn from official football players and Olympic athletes that placing a high priority on quality sleep is essential to high-level performance. It is never too late to change your sleeping habits. Those who believe sleep is "a waste of time" and takes away from productivity will likely suffer the long-term consequences of chronic disease and cognitive decline.

Sleep and Cancer

Extensive studies have revealed a causal relationship between lack of sleep and cancer risk. The risk of four different types of cancer (lung, ovarian, thyroid, and melanoma) appears to be increased in those individuals who exhibit inadequate sleep. In these human cohorts, sleep duration of less than five to six hours carries the highest risk. Rodent studies also identify an increased risk of malignancy with greater degrees of sleep deprivation.

The International Agency for Research on Cancer is a branch of the World Health Organization. It has declared that those who perform night shift work, including healthcare workers, airline pilots, and factory shift workers, are at higher risk for cancer. They have labeled night shift work as "probably carcinogenic to humans," with a higher risk of colorectal, prostate, and breast malignancies in this group. Likely, the disruption in the normal circadian rhythm of the human sleep cycle and the decrease in total and quality sleep duration are significant factors.

Healthy sleep habits might also be related to reduced cancer risk because melatonin helps regulate estrogen and growth hormone, two hormones known to contribute to various types of cancer. Melatonin appears to modify the estrogen-binding receptors on cells and potentially exerts a therapeutic benefit on both breast and prostate malignancies. Melatonin production is lower in shift workers and older patients, which may partially explain the higher incidence of malignancies in these patient populations. It also strengthens the argument that sleep deprivation can significantly increase the risk of some cancers.

Inflammation and Sleep

One fact I have consistently tried to hammer home throughout this book is that inflammation is a strong marker for chronic disease and reduction in survival. A 2015 study identified a correlation between elevated inflammatory markers and reduced survival in those individuals who slept less than six hours. As mentioned earlier, melatonin is a sleep hormone with an anti-inflammatory nature. Since these same inflammatory markers are seen in the presence of chronic diseases like hypertension, CHD, diabetes, and cancer, it would make sense that inadequate or ineffective melatonin levels would adversely affect these conditions and possibly cause decreased long-term survival.

On the other hand, good sleep quality has been associated with our body's capacity to reduce the inflammatory response that is provoked by infections. This factor appears to improve our ability to fight these infectious agents. Interferons are proteins that "interfere" with viral replication and help prevent the spread of viral infections in the body. Studies have revealed an increase in interferons in individuals with good-quality sleep. It is recognized that individuals with good sleep quality before vaccine reception have a heightened antibody response compared to those with inadequate or impaired sleep. It has also been identified that individuals with optimum sleep habits can have a severalfold reduction in the risk of viral infections compared to those with poor sleep hygiene.

Sleep Apnea

I would be remiss if I did not discuss one of the most frequent and potentially dangerous causes of sleep deprivation. Sleep apnea is a common disease that affects approximately 6–7 percent of the US population, and up to 50 percent of these patients are undiagnosed. African Americans are more than twice as likely to be diagnosed with sleep apnea compared to Caucasians. In addition, among men over forty, obesity and a large neck circumference of greater than sixteen inches are also significant risks. Oropharyngeal abnormalities such as chronic sinus or nasal obstruction, enlarged tonsils, or a small jaw size are also associated with sleep apnea. These observations can usually be detected with a good history and physical exam. However, I am still amazed by the many patients I see with characteristic features of this medical issue. "Seek, and you shall find."

The consequences of undetected sleep apnea can be enormous. Persistent hypertension, diabetes and insulin resistance, cardiovascular disease, and cardiac arrhythmias are some consequences of poorly treated or untreated sleep apnea. Cognitive dysfunction with memory issues is not uncommon. There is MRI evidence that decreased size of the memory-related mammillary bodies in the limbic system occurs with sleep apnea, and these memory issues may not be reversible.

What Can We Do?

An ever-expanding body of research points to the link between good sleep habits and improved longevity. Many of these good habits are simple and easy to implement, but bad habits die slowly. Two of the most challenging obstacles to overcome are guilt and lifestyle habits that prevent us from going to bed early. However, I cannot overemphasize how vital sleep duration and quality are to overall health. The following recommendations will lead you to good health and fantastic sleep.

Bedrooms should be dark and cool:

Deep sleep improves as the temperature decreases. Cooling mattresses (like Eight Sleep) or pads under a bed (like the Ooler system) can keep core body temperature low throughout the night and prevent wakefulness due to warming. These units can be expensive, but good sleep aids are precious investments, considering we should spend one-third of every twenty-four-hour day in bed. These systems can also benefit women who suffer from hot flashes at night. Failure to adequately allow our body to cool can significantly impact our ability to achieve deep sleep.

Blackout curtains are critical because melatonin release is delayed in the presence of all light. If you can't eliminate all light, you can use eye masks, which are effective and inexpensive.

Eliminate all screens:

Televisions, phones, tablets, and computers are blue-light-emitting devices that disrupt circadian rhythm. If you want to guarantee poor-quality sleep, watch TV before bed and keep checking your devices for messages and email. We are too connected, and our machines are addictive. They also disrupt our sleep and potentially shorten our lives. As has been noted many times, bedrooms are meant for two activities: sleeping and sexual intimacy. Turn off your devices and turn on the charm!

Develop a regular schedule:

Develop a schedule that allows for seven to eight hours of actual sleep. Setting a fixed time for bed and for arising in the morning is extremely important. Sleep efficiency is defined as the percentage of time asleep relative to the time in bed. For example, if you went to bed at 10:00 p.m. and arose at 6:00 a.m. but slept for 6.5 hours, your sleep efficiency would be approximately 85 percent. Sleep efficiency of 85 percent or greater is considered good. Although the value is reasonable, you cannot assume that you were in deep sleep or REM sleep the entire time you were asleep. Individuals with lower efficiency either spend too much time in bed or are restless at night. Many causes include higher core body temperature, alcohol excess, bladder issues, noise distractions, animals or children in bed, uneasy/snoring partners, and sleep apnea. All these causes are fixable with good discipline.

Do not spend too much time in bed awake:

If you can't sleep, leave the bedroom, and read a book or do some calming activity. Prayer or meditation are great relaxing tools late at night and are usually very effective at getting you back in bed. Phone apps that help with meditation and prayer are good as long as you keep the screen dark. Do not turn on the television or read on your phone or computer. Blue-light-blocking features on devices help somewhat, but any light will prolong the night and reduce sleep efficiency. This critical trap that so many insomniacs fall into leads to chronic sleep deprivation and true misery for many.

Make your bed off-limits for all sorts of creatures:

I am amazed at patients' guilt when they realize that their favorite dog or cat will have to sleep elsewhere. They will get over it! Children will rest better in their own beds and may even develop sleep issues if they can only sleep when sharing the bed with an adult. A snoring or restless partner may have sleep apnea. I remind my chronically fatigued patients that identifying sleep apnea can be lifesaving and treats two patients: the snorer and the snored-upon! I almost always ask the spouse of a suspected sleep apnea patient for their input. Invariably, those with sleep apnea think that they sleep soundly and don't know that they are slowly destroying their brain with repeated episodes of nightly hypoxia (low oxygen levels). I often find out that the spouse is sleeping in a separate bedroom.

Take some supplements that can help induce sleep:

Supplements, especially magnesium and melatonin, can help. I generally use magnesium threonate for my patients with sleep issues or nerve pain because it crosses the blood-brain barrier more quickly than other magnesium supplements. I usually do not recommend long-term melatonin, simply because it could suppress the body's natural melatonin production. A good walk in the early-morning sun can significantly increase our body's production of melatonin and assist with sleep induction later at night. Glycine is an amino acid that also improves sleep efficiency and quality in some patients. Phosphatidylserine works as a sleep enhancer by increasing the effect of serotonin and reducing the release of the stress hormone cortisol from the adrenal gland. This stress reduction reduces the barrier to sleep induction. Ashwagandha also appears to alleviate the impact of high cortisol levels that are caused by elevated stress. This therapeutic effect results in the alleviation of stress-mediated sleep induction in some individuals.

Don't eat food or drink alcohol immediately before bed:

You don't want to consume food before bed because it usually increases blood sugar, which compounds insulin resistance during sleep.

Alcohol is also a poor sleep-inducing agent and can be counterproductive because of its negative effect on REM sleep, sleep quality, and sleep efficiency. One should expect to "feel" the adverse impact of poor sleep whenever alcohol is used in excess. This impact can last several days if a drinking habit is not reversed.

Don't use regular over-the-counter medications:

Over-the-counter medications such as antihistamines shouldn't be used primarily as sleep aids. This suggestion includes the popular drug diphenhydramine. Although drowsiness is a side effect of this drug, the opposite reaction can occur in older patients. These individuals can develop agitation rather than sedation from certain antihistamines. This is clearly not a good thing, especially in demented patients. Additional side effects include urinary retention and constipation, which can be problems in older patients.

Use prescription sleep aids sparingly:

Benzodiazepines are a group of medications that are classified as sedative-hypnotics. These medications are commonly prescribed for insomnia and are beneficial for short-term sleep disturbances, but they are detrimental to long-term sleep because they can be addictive and are known to adversely affect REM sleep and deep sleep. Sadly, I have encountered many patients who have been on these medications for years and still experience significant sleep disturbances.

Understandably, some individuals may be hesitant to stop taking medications that they believe are helping them sleep, even when those medications are harming their sleep quality. Likely they are worried they won't be able to sleep. It's essential to approach these conversations with empathy and understanding, as fear of sleep deprivation can be a powerful motivator that can make individuals feel irrational or unyielding when medication withdrawal is recommended. We should encourage open and honest conversations with our patients about medication use and any concerns that individuals may have, and we should work together to find personalized treatment plans that balance the risks and benefits of medication use.

Adenosine and Caffeine

Adenosine is a naturally occurring chemical that is essential to brain activity. Its production increases during waking hours, provoking drowsiness as the day progresses. Adenosine's effect is modulated through four different adenosine receptors in the brain, and its effect is blocked by caffeine. As such, caffeine taken later in the day may make it more difficult for many individuals to fall asleep.

Interestingly, there may be a genetic component to how your body "clears" caffeine. The expression of a particular gene determines whether a specific caffeine-clearing enzyme works quickly or slowly. Fast metabolizers remove caffeine rapidly and don't seem to have any sleep disruption, even when caffeine is taken late in the day. Slow metabolizers have much more difficulty with caffeine clearance and can experience significant sleep induction and quality issues when caffeine is consumed after the morning. This caffeine-clearing enzyme is also affected by other factors. Food cooked at high temperature or chargrilled, cruciferous vegetables (broccoli, cauliflower, Brussels sprouts), and heavy exercise increase enzyme activity to clear caffeine more quickly. Grapefruit juice, carrots, celery, parsley, quercetin, and curcumin decrease enzyme activity and can prolong caffeine bioavailability. Smokers and women tend to clear the effects of caffeine more easily. Estrogen and nicotine enhance the liver enzyme that breaks down caffeine.

Slow metabolizers may be more susceptible to hypertension and heart rhythm abnormalities, although a recent analysis of several published studies in the journal *Circulation* did not identify a significantly enhanced risk of cardiovascular disease in those who drink less than five to six cups of coffee daily. In addition, caffeine consumption may reduce the risk of some cancers and may also reduce cognitive decline as well. So, while the overall message regarding caffeine is that it is safe and potentially beneficial for most people, still, it should be consumed early in the day to avoid any risk of sleep impairment. I also suggest that you pay attention to your body and your health. If caffeine makes you nervous or raises your heart rate or blood pressure, reduce, or eliminates it from your diet. If you absolutely cannot live without it, perhaps you can exercise or consume some cruciferous vegetables later in the day to enhance the caffeine-clearing enzyme activity in your body. This simple type of biohacking can have significant advantages for long-term health, considering the beneficial effects of caffeine on athletic performance and the value of exercise on longevity.

Takeaways

Sleep is an essential component of a healthy lifestyle—a forgotten soldier in the fight against chronic inflammatory diseases and enhanced cancer risk. Our previous concept of sleep deprivation as a sign of strength and toughness must be discarded and discouraged. Everyone should strive for seven to nine hours of sound, quality sleep to maximize health and longevity. In addition to a restful physical environment, spiritual enhancement using valuable ingredients like meditation, prayer, a virtuous lifestyle, and love of others can make our sleep both peaceful and restful.

1. Sleep is an essential and critical component of long-term health. There is a strong link between poor sleep and cardiovascular disease, many chronic diseases, and some cancers.
2. Critical factors to ensure adequate sleep include a cool and dark sleep environment, avoiding late-night screens, and avoiding excess alcohol.
3. Melatonin and other natural sleep aids can be used effectively in some instances. Prescription and over-the-counter medications are not good long-term choices and can lead to adverse outcomes.
4. The diagnosis and treatment of sleep apnea are critical to longevity.

Chapter 5

Dementia

The human face of dementia is often challenging to identify upon your first encounter. My initial recognition of this disease occurred in 1987, shortly after I had started practicing in a Chicago suburb. I first "met" Tim from the window of my automobile when driving home after late-night hospital rounds. He was always dressed in a suit and carried an attaché case that swung somewhat awkwardly as he walked slowly along the sidewalk. A dark fedora was always perched on his head. To outward appearances, he was a refined businessman returning home from a long workday. At first, I didn't seem to notice that he appeared to be talking to himself, nor did I perceive the partially untucked shirt and the uneven elements of his tie. I was much more focused on the illusion that he was a diligent and hardworking man that was providing support for his family. In a self-serving way, he inspired me as I worked late into the evenings.

    As the months passed, however, I became more aware of the fact that he seemed to be unaware of his surroundings. He would ignore streetlights until horns from oncoming cars startled him from his thoughts. I was perplexed that such an accomplished individual might be impaired, and I subconsciously refused to accept what my eyes and intuition told me. Everything finally came to clarity when I had a chance to meet with Tim at a local deli, and I realized that he was clearly impaired cognitively. I was crestfallen. I did not want to acknowledge that Tim was not the man I thought I knew. Deli workers told me Tim had long ago been dismissed from his workplace for declining performance. I learned that Tim had no close family to support him because his previous work habits had destroyed his family life. I learned valuable life lessons on that late summer evening that altered my perspective and gave me invaluable wisdom. I wrote about this experience in an essay titled "Driving Home with Tim."

Facts and Fundamentals

Dementia is a common disease, affecting far too many. The incidence of dementia worldwide is progressively increasing but appears to be decreasing in the United States and other developed countries. Yet despite this decrease, the prevalence of dementia is growing in the United States as the population ages. Incidence means the likelihood of getting a specific illness in a particular group. Prevalence, however, is the number of people with the illness.

For instance, if we talk about a specific type of cancer, incidence tells us how many people out of a certain number are expected to develop cancer within a specific time-frame, while prevalence tells us how many people already have cancer at a specific point in time. Understanding this difference can help us better understand the burden of a particular illness on a population, and it can help guide decisions about prevention and treatment efforts. If we do not adequately help reduce the risk of dementia, this prevalence will continue to burden the healthcare industry over the next thirty years and possibly far beyond.

Approximately six million people in the United States are living with some manifestation of Alzheimer's disease, a number that is expected to triple within the next thirty years. About one in ten Americans over sixty-five have Alzheimer's disease, and the current cost of care for these individuals approaches $300 billion. And those caring for family members with dementia are losing a lot of work time and income, and out-of-pocket expenses account for approximately 20 percent of annual expenditures for care. One can only imagine the overall costs of this disease in the future if current trends continue. Sadly, Alzheimer's disease is often progressive, with an average life expectancy of eight years once the diagnosis is established. In addition, there is no cure, and most current medications have limited benefits on the progression of clinical features. For this reason, you must take a proactive approach to your brain health early to prevent this devastating disease.

Genetics, including a gene called apolipoprotein E (APOE), can play a role in certain types of dementia, such as Alzheimer's. The APOE gene has different variants: APOE ε2, APOE ε3, and APOE ε4. The APOE ε4 variant increases the risk of developing late-onset Alzheimer's disease. However, it's important to note that having this gene variant does not guarantee that a person will develop the disease, and not having it does not guarantee protection. Many other factors, including lifestyle and environment, also contribute to the risk of developing dementia.

With that said, familial Alzheimer's disease accounts for a small percentage of all cases. Most Alzheimer's cases are sporadic, with more complex and less deterministic genetic factors. Genetic risk factors, such as the APOE gene, can increase the susceptibility to late-onset Alzheimer's disease, but they do not guarantee its development. It may benefit individuals to obtain genetic testing if they are concerned about a family history of early-onset dementia so appropriate preventative and proactive steps can be started.

Fortunately, many risk factors for developing Alzheimer's are modifiable or preventable.

Some of these include:

- lower educational status
- Diabetes
- Hypertension
- lipid abnormalities
- Smoking
- Inactivity
- Depression
- social isolation
- traumatic head injury
- sleep apnea

Age is the most significant nonmodifiable risk, but many other factors are modifiable or preventable. Although lower educational status may be considered a nonmodifiable risk, education can be a lifelong experience, even when educational opportunities have been limited in early life. Traumatic brain injury is preventable, but there is a clearly increased risk of dementia after the injury has occurred.

Insulin resistance, another risk factor that can often be modified, is linked to cognitive decline, and this metabolic dysfunction is strongly linked to obesity, a sedentary lifestyle, and diabetes. It is known that lifestyle changes that reduce insulin resistance (calorie restriction, regular exercise, weight loss) also positively impact cognitive decline later in life. Therefore, it should not be surprising that lifestyle adjustments can benefit late-life mental status and even alter the trajectory of early-onset Alzheimer's disease if implemented effectively.

The long-term incidence of Alzheimer's dementia is especially concerning given the upsurge in childhood and adult obesity over the last three decades. The prevalence of obesity in US children up to age nineteen years is over 20 percent, while the adult prevalence exceeds 42 percent. These statistics are staggering! A higher body mass index (BMI) is associated with an enhanced risk of hypertension, diabetes, and abnormal lipids. Despite the recent evidence of a reduction in the incidence of Alzheimer's disease in the United States and other advanced countries, the dramatic uptick in obesity and diabetes over the past thirty years suggests that the metabolic abnormalities common to these issues will lead to a rebound increase in Alzheimer's disease.

Remember that almost 75 percent of the US adult population (age twenty years and above) is clinically overweight. Even though there has been dramatic advancement in treating lipid abnormalities, heart disease, and hypertension over the past few decades, optimizing these risk factors in patients remains challenging. Many hypertensive patients are sub optimally treated, and a significant percentage of adult patients' manifest noncompliance with diet and drug strategies for these risk factors. This must change if we are going to make any progression in the control of dementia in the future.

Another concern regarding cognitive decline and lifestyle habits is exposure to excess screen time from computers, tablets, and phones. Three studies have linked moderate to high television exposure with brain gray matter loss. The authors of these studies link this relationship to a sedentary lifestyle, which may be true. Interestingly, a recent study on fruit flies revealed an increase of brain degeneration with daily exposure to blue light. This study raises the question of whether high levels of prolonged exposure to computers, television, and phone screens contribute to subtle brain injury. Of course, we are not fruit flies, and direct scientific links may not be entirely acceptable. Still, the damaging effects of blue light exposure on these tiny insects caused premature aging of their brains and retinal degeneration. This latest study also correlates with earlier studies from mice and should not be dismissed by those who have prolonged exposure to blue light from screens.

In addition, evidence shows that factors for early-life cardiac risk are also associated with a significant increase in cognitive decline later in life. Individuals with associated cardiovascular risk factors such as high blood pressure, diabetes, elevated lipids, and long-term cigarette use can also develop vascular disease in the arteries of the brain. These changes can lead to a less frequent cause of memory decline known as vascular dementia. The differentiation between vascular dementia and Alzheimer's disease can be subtle and difficult to differentiate. Unfortunately, the outcomes are not significantly altered long term unless aggressive lifestyle changes are instituted earlier in life.

Underlying Pathology

Nonmedical individuals might not feel they need to understand all the complexities happening inside the body in response to a certain disease. Alzheimer's disease, however, is interesting because the possible underlying changes in the brain may have motivational consequences if one focuses on reducing the risks. In addition, currently prevailing theories about the causes of Alzheimer's give some hope regarding early diagnosis, prevention, and treatment. That said, please remember that Alzheimer's disease is not curable and can be very difficult to treat when it develops. For this reason, taking active measures throughout life to reduce risk is imperative.

Two main areas of the brain are affected by Alzheimer's disease. The hippocampus is part of the lower brain and is primarily responsible for forming short- and long-term memory and managing overall spatial orientation in our world. Patients with Alzheimer's disease struggle with recent memory loss and may become confused about their location. It is common for these patients to get lost or need clarification in unfamiliar environments. Interestingly, long-term memory can be preserved, suggesting that the hippocampus has "offloaded" some of its memories into other brain areas for storage. Patients with Alzheimer's can frequently get confused about recent memory issues, but they may be able to remember things from their childhood and early work activities. They may also be able to find their way home if they can locate familiar landmarks from their past.

I have seen many patients with cognitive issues that become acutely confused and agitated when hospitalized and surrounded by unfamiliar caretakers. One common reason that hospital stays are prolonged is confusion and agitation in cognitively impaired patients. Families fear taking these patients home when they are uncooperative or confused even when their underlying medical issue that initially prompted the admission has been treated. In addition, a standard but sad resolution to this problem is to transfer a patient to a nursing home, which requires time and longer hospitalization. Early discharge to a familiar environment can often "cure" the agitation and confusion, but in my experience, it is tough to convince families of its merit.

The second main area of the brain impacted by Alzheimer's is the neocortex, the higher part of the brain that is involved with comprehension, emotion, and memory.

It is the most significant part of our cerebral cortex and critically affects many areas:

- our ability to comprehend input from external sources
- language development, spatial orientation, and reasoning
- simple and complex learning tasks

It should come as no surprise that individuals with Alzheimer's disease struggle with complex logic and learning and may have associative problems with speech. Furthermore, the neocortex plays a significant role in sleep. It is common for patients with progressive cognitive decline to have significant sleep-related issues, further propagating cognitive decline. Aggression and anger can ensue as a rather alarming personality change when sleep deprivation progresses.

One of the things that makes Alzheimer's such a tragic disease is that when an individual begins to demonstrate memory issues and difficulties with reasoning, degenerative changes have already happened within the hippocampus and the neocortex. These changes generally develop slowly, even over decades, and drug treatment strategies tend only to stabilize or slow their progression. Prevention and early intervention remain the primary goals of treatment before advanced and potentially irreversible damage ensues.

There are a few ideas about why people get Alzheimer's disease. One idea is that when a protein in the brain breaks down, it can build up around cells and cause inflammation, which damages brain cells. Another idea is that another protein in the brain can twist and create tangles, which also harm brain cells. A third idea is that over time, our body can get stressed by chemicals that are produced naturally in our cells. This stress can cause damage to our brain and other organs, and it's called oxidative stress. The brain is especially vulnerable to this type of damage because it needs a lot of oxygen to function properly. When our brain cells don't work well, it can lead to memory and thinking problems like in Alzheimer's disease.

To understand the process of aging in the brain and other organ systems, it is helpful to explain this concept of oxidative stress. In simple terms, "oxidative" refers to a process that involves adding oxygen or losing electrons from molecules. It often leads to chemical reactions in the cell where molecules combine with oxygen or experience changes in their electrical charge. In the context of oxidative stress, there is an excess of harmful molecules, called free radicals or reactive oxygen species (ROS), which can damage cells and DNA by taking electrons from other molecules. This damage is often caused by free radicals "stealing" electrons from these molecules, disrupting their normal functioning.

The body has natural defense mechanisms to neutralize free radicals, such as antioxidants, which can donate electrons to stabilize the free radicals and prevent their harmful effects. However, when there is an overwhelming number of free radicals or a deficiency of antioxidants, the balance is disrupted, and oxidative stress can occur. These free radicals have good and bad effects on other cellular systems. For example, they can occasionally help to fight off infections in the body. Still, they are more often harmful to mitochondrial function if they are not neutralized by antioxidants. Antioxidants "give" an additional electron to the ROS, making them much less toxic to our cells.

An ongoing balance needs to occur within our cells to clear out the ROS and reduce the toxicity of these particles. An abundance of antioxidants enables cells to fight off aging and mitochondrial degeneration. Please remember that intracellular mitochondria are the engines that drive the overall function and health of each of our cells, including the brain, heart, liver, and other vital organs. Any imbalance between excess ROS production or low antioxidant availability is known as oxidative stress and can create a toxic and potentially destructive cascade that leads to cell degeneration or death.

The brain has extremely high oxygen demands and is particularly susceptible to oxidative damage. The progressive loss of mitochondrial function and efficiency secondary to oxidative stress in brain cells may significantly contribute to cognitive decline. More importantly, Alzheimer's disease has recently been considered a manifestation of a more diffuse aging process related to mitochondrial deterioration. This concept is known as the mitochondrial cascade theory, which suggests that mitochondrial decline in many organ systems results from chronic inflammation and inadequate bioavailable antioxidants. This progressive deterioration in the internal engine (mitochondria) leads to cellular aging and death. Based on this theory, enhanced intake of antioxidants in foods and other sources of cellular preservation, such as exercise, have been studied to better assess if alterations in lifestyle can reduce or delay cognitive decline.

Doctors use different ways to figure out if someone has Alzheimer's disease, like testing their memory and doing brain scans. Some types of scans can see if there are harmful proteins in the brain that might cause Alzheimer's disease. These scans can sometimes provide information regarding the extent and stage of the disease in the brain. There's also research about whether things like eating healthy foods or exercising can help slow down the process of cognitive decline.

But most of the time, healthcare providers will ask the patient questions and do memory tests to see if they have any problems remembering things.

Genetic testing can also be a valuable tool for detecting inherited markers for Alzheimer's disease. Although valuable in determining risk, these markers cannot predict that an individual will develop Alzheimer's disease later in life. Their value lies in providing a risk factor in the same way that smoking, hypertension, and diabetes enhance the risk of this disease. These gene markers can (and should) serve as a strong motivation to make corrective lifestyle adjustments that can slow the development and progression of dementia. A proactive approach early in adulthood could profoundly affect later-life health and happiness.

Prevention Options

Paul Allen, one of the founders of Microsoft, was actively involved in investigating Alzheimer's disease through his philanthropy. The Allen Institute has been a source of valuable research in attempting to discover effective treatments for this disease. Reflecting on these frustrations, he said, "Everyone's dream is to take a pill-take a pill every day so that you won't have Alzheimer's." In the end, however, there is no pill. There is no simple treatment. There is no effective cure once the disease has taken hold of one's life.

The path toward Alzheimer's begins many years before its outward manifestations. The disease is insidious at onset, but the framework is frequently set through bad habits and poor lifestyles. I don't chastise patients for making previous poor choices because we are all periodically guilty of poor eating habits and sedentary lifestyles. Instead, I encourage them to take up a new "mantle" of health that will reap benefits in the struggle against cognitive decline. It is fundamental to this process to remind my patients that dementia is most often progressive and largely untreatable when symptoms ensue. So, you don't have time to waste.

Several proposed medication treatments are for the established diagnosis of Alzheimer's dementia. The currently prescribed medications focus on the two most important neurotransmitters in the brain: acetylcholine (ACh) and glutamate. Both chemicals are essential for signal transmission between brain cells (neurons). They play a vital role in human learning and memory development, and any imbalance or decrease in the availability of these chemicals can lead to cognitive decline. In addition, they allow the transmission of messaging between cells through a gap in the neurons known as the synaptic junction. This junction is the location where brain cells connect and share information. Both glutamate and ACh are essential to this transmission.

Medications that inhibit the degradation of ACh at the synaptic junction increase the available amount of ACh. These agents are called acetylcholinesterase inhibitors. These medications may increase memory in early and moderately impaired patients, but the response is variable. Three drugs are currently available for clinical use: galantamine, donepezil, and rivastigmine. They have varying results, but their use is limited by nausea, vomiting, and other gastrointestinal side effects.

Glutamate availability is a double-edged sword in the brain. It is essential to have high levels of this chemical within the synaptic junction. Still, excess glutamate along the cell surface in the non-synaptic area of the cell leads to overexcitability of the neuron and eventual cell death. Memantine is a drug that appears to block excess glutamate in this non-synaptic region selectively and reduces neuron cell death. It is not a good choice for early dementia and is frequently used as an add-on to other ACh-blocking drugs. However, GI side effects, headaches, and worsening confusion limit its use.

A new monoclonal antibody named aducanumab has just received FDA approval to treat mild cognitive impairment, but it is still subject to controversy. It appears to reduce the beta-amyloid in the brain of these patients, but there is no overwhelming evidence of significant improvement in treated patients. Furthermore, the drug must be administered intravenously, and up to 40 percent of treated patients develop brain swelling while on treatment. Remarkably, the FDA approved the drug despite their advisory panel overwhelmingly recommending against this decision. Several panelists resigned over this move. In addition, the drug costs approximately $56,000 per year.

Medicare is set to cover the cost of this drug, but the co-pay may be significant for some patients. To put this in perspective, it would cost Medicare over $168 billion annually to cover half of the current patients (three million) diagnosed with Alzheimer's disease. Given that the total Medicare budget for fiscal year 2019 was $644 billion, this very questionable drug would cost over 25 percent of the entire Medicare budget each year!

I realize that Alzheimer's disease is devastating and incurable, but aducanumab is the perfect example of medicine gone wrong. As physicians, we are given a costly drug option that has not been proved beneficial. The side effects are significant, and the delivery route requires medical supervision. In addition, it may take an additional ten years before we know if phase 4 clinical trials reveal clear benefits. This is crazy! Therefore, prevention is of paramount importance. The overall cost of a healthy diet, regular exercise, and good sleep is minuscule, but I cannot seem to create a pill that provides good self-discipline and motivation. I can only warn my patients that the potential cost of dementia is far beyond the value of the medicines. The progressive loss of independence and the declining memory can never be replaced. In addition, the burden on loved ones can produce a sense of guilt and depression that destroys the remaining "golden years."

Statin therapy has been proposed as a treatment option for dementia as a preventative agent. Although initial reports were optimistic, the long-term benefits do not support this treatment. A very detailed review from the Cochrane Group reveals the lack of benefits of statins in dementia prevention. There have also been some concerns about whether statin therapy worsens cognition, but most recent studies do not support this possibility. However, there is some evidence that visual-spatial function may be adversely affected in elderly patients with statin-induced low cholesterol. This function is essential for three-dimensional spatial recognition in daily movement and driving. My approach regarding statin therapy in dementia prevention and treatment is simple: I don't use statins because there is no clear evidence of benefit, and there is some evidence of potential harm in some patients. Suppose there is any question that statin therapy may contribute to memory or confusion. In that case, I suggest a brief drug "holiday" of two to three weeks to determine if there is any cognitive improvement from this therapy.

The average retirement age in the United States is sixty-three to sixty-five years. Tragically, approximately 10 percent of this age group will already have developed Alzheimer's dementia. This number doubles every ten years in age, so over 30–35 percent of individuals over eighty-five will have some cognitive impairment.

Undeniably, embracing preventative measures can significantly improve our health as we age. However, it is crucial to approach this topic with empathy and understanding, acknowledging that various factors influence lifestyle choices. Breaking free from long-standing habits can be an uphill battle for many individuals.

Instead of assigning blame, fostering a supportive environment that allows individuals to make positive choices for their well-being is essential. By raising awareness, providing education, and offering accessible resources, we can inspire and guide people toward healthier lifestyles. For most of us, change is a gradual process, unique to everyone. Therefore, we must be patient and understanding, recognizing that it takes time to make significant adjustments. By instilling a sense of optimism and encouraging personal growth, physicians can motivate individuals to explore new challenges, develop new skills, and embrace habits that contribute to their overall health and happiness. We do not have to become victims of our indulgences. We can cultivate a culture of well-being for ourselves and others that allows us to focus on a healthier and more fulfilling life.

The best approach to reduce your risk of cognitive decline in general, and Alzheimer's disease specifically, is to focus on prevention and lifestyle changes. Consuming a healthy and vitamin-enriched diet that includes vitamins E, C, and B (especially B6 and B12) is integral to this approach. In addition, optimizing the intake of omega-3 fatty acids, zinc, and vitamin D3 will move the needle significantly in your favor. Daily exercise, plenty of sunshine (at least forty-five minutes daily if possible), excellent sleep habits, and avoidance of smoking and excess alcohol are inexpensive ways of protecting yourself against slow and progressive intellectual decline. These practices are relatively easy to implement and should be introduced as soon as possible if you want to protect your mind and body.

Diet remains an essential and integral component of treating all inflammatory diseases, including cognitive issues. The Mediterranean and DASH diets are good starting points, but the MIND (Mediterranean-DASH Intervention for Neurodegenerative

Delay) diet combines the two and has become one of the preeminent diets for preventing and treating cognitive decline.

The MIND diet was developed to promote brain health and reduce the risk of cognitive decline and dementia. The diet emphasizes consuming nutrient-dense, plant-based foods, such as leafy greens, berries, nuts, and beans, while limiting the intake of processed and high-fat foods.

- Berries are rich in antioxidants, which help protect the brain from oxidative stress and inflammation, which are thought to contribute to cognitive decline.
- Leafy greens, such as spinach and kale, are rich in vitamins and minerals, including vitamin K and folate, linked to improved cognitive function.
- Nuts are a good source of healthy fats, fiber, and vitamin E, which may help reduce inflammation and protect against cognitive decline.
- Whole grains are a good source of fiber, linked to better cognitive function, and provide essential vitamins and minerals that may support brain health.
- Fatty fish, such as salmon, are rich in omega-3 fatty acids, which are important for brain health and have been linked to a reduced risk of cognitive decline and dementia.
- Poultry, such as chicken and turkey, is included in the MIND diet as a lean protein source, as it is lower in saturated fat than red meat. While it is not as prominently featured as other foods on the MIND diet (such as leafy greens, berries, and nuts), poultry is considered a healthy protein source that can be part of a balanced diet.
- Olive oil has a high content of monounsaturated fats, polyunsaturated fats, and polyphenols. Polyphenols are plant compounds that appear to have both anti-inflammatory and antioxidant benefits. These components of olive oil have

been shown in observational studies to protect against cognitive decline.

Overall, the MIND diet emphasizes whole, nutrient-dense foods rich in vitamins, minerals, and antioxidants linked to improved brain health. By limiting processed and high-fat foods, the diet may also help reduce inflammation, which is thought to contribute to cognitive decline. Enhanced intake of foods high in flavonoids has also been shown to decrease the risk of cognitive decline.

Foods with a high flavonoid content include:

- some herbs and spices (parsley, oregano, and saffron)
- dark chocolate
- Tea
- berries (those with the highest flavonoid content include acai, elderberry, blackberry, and blueberry)
- Kale
- Onions
- Capers
- Radishes
- red cabbage
- small amounts of red wine
- some tree fruits (plums, pears, and apples)

You can see that almost everyone will find a few of these whole food sources easy to add to their daily intake to enhance their brain power!

Calorie restriction also appears to benefit memory preservation for overweight individuals. One study revealed significant memory benefits with a 30 percent reduction in daily calories. In addition, this approach likely reduces the pro-inflammatory effects of elevated blood sugar and the negative consequences of hypertension on brain neuroplasticity.

Coffee intake has been associated with reducing dementia and Parkinson's disease. However, it is uncertain if quercetin, the antioxidant in coffee beans, is the primary reason for this benefit. Still, a simple thing such as enjoying a few cups of coffee can provide long-term benefits to overall brain health. It is also feasible that the polyphenols in caffeine help activate the antiaging process whereby our older cellular components, like mitochondria and ribosomes, are recycled for new and healthier cellular elements.

Even late in life, regular exercise appears to have clear advantages on cognition. Many animal and human studies have identified the benefits of moderate to high physical activity on brain health. The exact biologic cause is not settled, but regular (preferably daily) exercise has been shown to increase brain blood flow. In addition, regular exercise appears to lead to enhanced neuroplasticity. This term is an exciting concept that identifies the actual capacity of the brain to develop new neurons, synapses, and blood vessels in response to enhanced physical activity. This means the brain can continue growing and repairing itself if provided with increased blood flow and hormonal stimulants. By committing to regular exercise throughout your life, you have a powerful and affordable tool to protect your brain health. So, how much do you value your brain? This question becomes increasingly important as we age and can motivate us to prioritize exercise in our daily routines.

Supplements

Supplements retain a role in treating Alzheimer's and other forms of dementia. Still, the data is somewhat conflicting, and many critics decry the random use of these treatments as false or misleading science. My approach is different. Alzheimer's dementia is not curable and is often progressive and devastating to both the patient and their family. So, choosing certain supplements that are safe, effective, and inexpensive offers an effective alternative for patients and families who are looking for ways to improve the trajectory of this disease.

Elevated homocysteine levels have been causally related to several medical issues, including increased vascular damage, blood clotting risk, and possibly enhanced stroke risk. Notably, there appears to be a potential twofold increased risk of Alzheimer's dementia in patients with elevated homocysteine levels.

I should state here that I am focusing on some supplements that do not have clear scientific benefits but have a beneficial effect on oxidative stress. Since oxidative stress causes mitochondrial damage and antioxidants combat this damage, I am optimistic that these nutritional supplements can have a salutary benefit on a disease (Alzheimer's) with no current cure.

Vitamin B:

Some individuals have a deficiency of B vitamins such as B6, B12, and folic acid. Adding these supplements can be an effective tool in normalizing elevated homocysteine values. These levels can also be reduced by lowering protein intake and consuming more fruits and vegetables that contain high B vitamins, including folic acid, B6, and B12. Leafy vegetables, beans, and oranges are good starting points to treat elevated homocysteine levels. B vitamin supplements are also reasonable for people at higher risk or those with elevated homocysteine levels. Folic acid may improve cognitive function in patients with elevated homocysteine levels.

Vitamin D3:

Most elderly patients have low vitamin D3, especially when daylight hours are short. African Americans are especially susceptible to this vitamin depletion. There appears to be a causal link between vitamin D deficiency and the development of Alzheimer's disease, and supplementation seems practical and appropriate. I recommend a daily vitamin D3 dose of 5000 IU for most patients.

Vitamin E:

While vitamin E has been extensively studied in preventing and treating Alzheimer's disease, the data is conflicting. It is believed to have some benefits based on its antioxidant properties. Vitamin E is a fat-soluble vitamin that has eight different components. Even in high doses, selective supplementation has not been shown to clearly alter the course of cognitive decline. However, it is an antioxidant whose primary role is to protect cells from the damage caused by free radicals. This effect reduces the risk of damaging oxidative stress, and this benefit may be additive when coupled with other antioxidants. Nuts and seeds (sunflower, almonds, pine nuts), fish, avocado, and even natural peanut butter are excellent dietary sources of this valuable vitamin. Wheat germ oil is the richest source of vitamin E and can be added to daily foods.

Herbs and oils:

These can sometimes be used to treat cognitive decline, especially Bacopa monnieri, turmeric, and sage. In addition, these agents have demonstrated anti-inflammatory effects in laboratory studies, and sage improves cognition in humans likely through a positive effect on the neurotransmitter acetylcholine. The overall effects are somewhat limited, but even small incremental benefits can add up for the long-term treatment of Alzheimer's.

Gotu kola is an herb that has anti-inflammatory properties. It has been used to treat cognitive decline in poststroke patients and those with mild cognitive impairment and can benefit cognitive function for these patients.

Quercetin:

Quercetin is a natural plant pigment and powerful antioxidant found in the skin of many fruits, vegetables, and grains. As a natural antioxidant, it helps combat the effects of free radicals and reduces inflammation throughout the body. Its antioxidant benefits may have a role in reducing cognitive decline in individuals with a higher risk of ongoing inflammatory damage within the neurons.

Growth hormone (GH) supplementation:

Recently there has been much interest in GH supplementation, especially in older individuals. For this reason, it is essential to address this issue as it relates to cognition and life extension. There is a close interplay between GH and another growth-like hormone called IGF-1.

IGF-1, which stands for insulin-like growth factor 1, is a protein hormone that plays a crucial role in growth and development. GH is produced and secreted by the pituitary gland; a small gland located at the base of the brain. Its primary function is stimulating growth in various tissues and organs throughout the body. GH secretion is regulated by a complex feedback system involving the hypothalamus, which releases growth hormone-releasing hormone (GHRH) to stimulate GH production, and somatostatin, which inhibits GH release. Once GH is released into the bloodstream, it travels to target tissues and stimulates the production and secretion of IGF-1 by the liver and other tissues. IGF-1 acts as the primary mediator of GH's growth-promoting effects, such as skeletal and muscle growth, organ development, and overall body growth early in life. It regulates metabolism, enhances protein synthesis, and promotes tissue repair and regeneration.

It binds to specific receptors on target cells, triggering a cascade of cellular responses that promote cell growth, replication, and differentiation.

The problem is low IGF-1 levels in nonhuman studies (worms and mice) extend longevity by 40–50 percent! That is probably why GH supplements may be a double-edged sword in later life— they enhance functionality but do not prolong life. So, what are we to do? We are not worms or mice, so the correlation is not infallible but can be very confusing. The most important message is that very low and very high IGF-1 levels should be avoided.

But there are strong reasons to consider enhancing IGF-1 availability.

Positives of IGF-1:

1. Growth and development: IGF-1 is essential for normal growth and development, particularly during childhood and adolescence. It promotes skeletal and muscle growth, organ development, and overall body growth.
2. Tissue repair and regeneration: The hormone is crucial in tissue repair and regeneration. It helps heal injuries, including wounds and fractures, by stimulating cell proliferation and promoting the synthesis of new proteins.
3. Metabolism regulation: IGF-1 regulates metabolism, including the metabolism of glucose, proteins, and fats. It helps maintain stable blood sugar levels and supports energy production.
4. Cognitive function: This hormone has been linked to cognitive function and brain health. Adequate levels of IGF-1 are essential for normal brain development and function, and deficiencies in IGF-1 have been associated with cognitive impairments.

Negatives of IGF-1:

1. Overgrowth disorders: Excess levels of IGF-1 can lead to overgrowth disorders, such as acromegaly in adults and gigantism in children. These conditions result in abnormal growth of bones, tissues, and organs, which can cause various health problems.
2. Cancer risk: Elevated levels of IGF-1 have been associated with an increased risk of certain cancers, including breast, prostate, and colorectal cancers. However, the relationship between IGF-1 and cancer is complex and still under investigation.
3. Insulin resistance: High levels of IGF-1 can contribute to insulin resistance, a condition where cells become less responsive to the effects of insulin, leading to impaired glucose metabolism and an increased risk of type 2 diabetes. This effect appears to occur because insulin and IGF-1 share similarities in their structure and function. High levels of IGF-1 may lead to confusion at the insulin receptor. In addition, IGF-1 can promote the production of inflammatory substances (cytokines) that also impair insulin signaling and can lead to the adverse effects of insulin resistance.

The best ways to temporarily increase IGF-1 naturally include strenuous exercise and weight training. Thirty minutes of sauna therapy also appears to increase IGF-1 and reduce cardiovascular mortality in older men. Altering our gene expression with healthy polyphenols and other foods (berries, green tea, turmeric, and dark chocolate) helps our bodies adjust to the harmful effects of oxidative stress induced by poor diet and other factors. The benefit of this IGF-1 regulation appears to reduce inflammatory cytokines and allows for an enhancement of the previously mentioned neuroplasticity. Increasing neuron repair and new growth can have significant benefits on long-term cognition.

IGF-1 levels can be significantly reduced with fasting, and multiple studies have revealed the benefits of either time-restricted eating (eating within a six- to eight-hour window) or intermittent fasting of twenty-four to seventy-two hours. This approach allows IGF-1 levels to fall significantly, leading to cellular repair and extension of cellular life. It is unclear what constitutes the best duration of fasting, but there appear to be benefits across multiple different fasting strategies. The use of fasting seems more significant than calorie restriction alone, even though weight reduction from reduced calorie intake is expected during various fasting or time-restricted eating protocols. The time-restricted eating approach has been very successful in my practice, and patients seem to embrace this strategy long term because it is simple to implement.

There appears to be even more significant motivation when they recognize the proactive benefits of reducing cognitive decline. Restricting one's food consumption to a six- to eight-hour window (noon until post-dinner) is an attainable goal for most of my patients. The elimination of late-night snacking and early-morning sugar consumption (cereal, donuts, sweetened coffee) allows the body to use up its glycogen stores and transition to burning fat. The addition of early-morning exercise can further enhance the lack of sugar storage and promote the induction of fat breakdown. This transition can take several days and be challenging, but it is worth the suffering. The objective of driving down fasting insulin levels is to promote a beneficial effect on fat metabolism by removing the suppressive effect of high circulating insulin levels on lipolysis. This effect uses stored fat as a primary energy source and allows for the benefit of ketone bodies (breakdown products of fat metabolism) to fuel brain energy.

Short-term reduction in IGF-1 levels correlates with a drop in insulin levels that occurs with fasting protocols, but more extreme and prolonged fasting protocols (days or weeks) cause IGF-1 levels to become too low and can result in decreased muscle mass, decreased bone density, and delayed tissue repair.

Caution About the Ketogenic Diet

The importance of a reduced carbohydrate diet and a ketogenic diet for treating various forms of cognitive impairment has recently gained traction. The effect of a ketogenic-type diet in these patients appears to reduce brain cellular inflammation through different cellular adaptive mechanisms. In addition, in some studies, this diet seems neuroprotective against further cell loss and can improve mitochondrial function. One of the current theories regarding the onset of dementia is related to increased insulin resistance. As we age, the brain's ability to utilize sugar decreases, resulting in reduced energy availability for cellular growth and sustenance. This transition appears to lead to mitochondrial degeneration and neurodegeneration. Brain cells can be literally "starved" because of the inability to obtain adequate energy. Ketone bodies easily cross the brain barrier and are an excellent alternative energy source.

Although the benefits of a ketogenic diet sound inviting, I cannot be a strong advocate for this long-term dietary approach because it can be very challenging to follow properly. In addition, limiting fruits and vegetables reduces many of the beneficial nutrients in these foods and may have a counterproductive effect. The risk of liver issues, kidney stones, and cardiovascular disease in older individuals appears to be increased and cannot be ignored. Patients with cognitive issues may not cooperate with spouses or partners in their willingness to adhere to this diet. I have learned that it is a significant obstacle for my patients and families when a cognitively impaired individual fails to understand the value of a significant change in their lifelong diet pattern. I am much more inclined to suggest a diet that helps to lower the number of processed foods and simple sugars.

Medium-chain triglycerides (MCTs) are triglyceride-rich fats that are easily absorbable and can cross the blood-brain barrier.

They can also be easily broken down into ketones, an excellent source of immediate energy for our brains. Supplementing with these products in patients with cognitive impairment has been shown to improve cognition in some short-term studies and may be a good option for long-term treatment. However, monitoring for excess ketone production in certain patients with diabetes, dehydration, and other medical issues is essential.

Role of BDNF

Brain-derived neurotrophic factor (BDNF) is a signaling protein that may act as a hormone for various critical processes in our brain. Without getting into the science, understand that you want higher levels of BDNF as you age to prevent cognitive decline. How can you accomplish this goal? I return to my reliable favorites for health and longevity: exercise and calorie restriction, especially a lower carbohydrate intake. Aerobic exercise and specially coordinated movement-related activities like dance enhance BDNF levels and improve cognitive function in early dementia. I am hopeful that integrated sports such as tennis (including table tennis) and the new fad of pickleball will serve as conduits for reducing cognitive decline in our aging population. It is essential to emphasize. However, exercising with good eating and sleep habits will maintain the overall benefit. A combination of lifestyle changes offers the best option for healthy brain aging.

In addition to good lifestyle habits like aerobic exercise and weight maintenance, certain supplements such as lion's mane and omega-3 fish oil can increase BDNF levels. Lactobacillus plantarum probiotic supplements also appear to offer benefits, and this effect points out the link between the brain and the gut. Good gut health is critical to good brain function!

Low BDNF levels are also noted in depression and anxiety, common findings in the elderly and those with early cognitive decline. The same lifestyle and dietary recommendations apply. Interestingly, those with PTSD also appear to benefit from treatments that enhance BDNF levels. Remember that our brain can always grow and reorganize itself (neuroplasticity), so never give up trying ways to improve your brain health. It is worth it!

All the supplements worldwide will only benefit you if you maintain a healthy and nutritious diet. I will again emphasize an important concept I often repeat to my patients: You can NEVER out-supplement or out-exercise a bad diet. Do not spend excessive money on supplements on the false premise that they will overcome your nutritional failures. There is an endless list of so-called health gurus who want you to believe that their supplements will melt away fat while you sleep. If it seems too good to be true, it is! As with much in life, self-discipline and strong effort are the pathways to success. There are very few shortcuts to health that provide sustained benefits. Don't be fooled, and you will enjoy the victory of good health in the long run.

Takeaways

1. The prevalence of dementia is increasing in the United States and will significantly impact healthcare expenditures over the next several decades.
2. Age is the most significant risk factor, but insulin resistance, inactivity, head trauma, and hypertension are some of the more common contributors to dementia.
3. The hippocampus and the neocortex are involved with memory and other critical brain functions and are most affected by Alzheimer's dementia.
4. The onset of symptoms is a late manifestation of the disease and signifies the need for early preventative measures in higher-risk individuals.
5. Alzheimer's dementia is one of the only significant diseases

with no cure.
6. A detailed and complete evaluation of all patients with memory loss is warranted to exclude other treatable illnesses. There are some diseases that mimic dementia and can be effectively treated and occasionally "cured" with proper diagnosis.
7. Drug therapies have limited benefits, ongoing side effects, and cost issues.
8. Lifestyle changes can significantly positively impact the incidence and progression of Alzheimer's disease.
9. Dietary adjustments may offer a beneficial role in Alzheimer's treatment and should be tried.
10. Targeted supplements may also have a role in altering the course of patients with cognitive decline.

Chapter 6

Preventing the Top Five Causes of Death

"Medicine aims to prevent disease and prolong life; the ideal of medicine is to eliminate the need of a physician."

William J. Mayo

In the late spring of 1981, I found myself in San Francisco for interviews related to a possible fellowship in critical care medicine. As an internal medicine resident, I was drawn to the excitement and the challenge of ICU care. I loved caring for critically ill patients. I reveled in bedside procedures such as intubation, placing large-bore catheters into patients' hearts and large veins, and treating low blood pressure, severe infections, and acute heart and lung ailments. I felt that ICU care was at the sharp end of the spear in medical care, and I wanted to be on the very end of the tip.

At that time, San Francisco had some top-tier fellowship programs. I had received special permission from my cardiology fellowship director to delay starting my fellowship in cardiology for one year while engaged in critical care training.

As I walked around San Francisco after completing my interview process, I experienced two different thoughts:

1. It is cold in San Francisco! As a midwestern native, I always expected California to be hot and balmy, and I had packed my clothes accordingly. I smiled when I read the quote (falsely attributed to Mark Twain): "The coldest winter I ever saw was the summer I spent in San Francisco."
2. Many young men had occupied most of the intensive care beds in the two hospitals where I'd participated in early-morning medical rounds. These young men suffered from severe respiratory illness, and many had already been placed on ventilators to assist with oxygenation and breathing. It was clear from the bedside that these individuals were gravely ill. What was even more concerning, however, was that none of the expert critical care specialists had any idea why they were so sick and what was causing such a life-threatening illness in previously healthy men.

Soon after my return, the *Morbidity and Mortality Weekly Report* published the first cases of pneumocystis carinii pneumonia in its June 5, 1981, report. All five patients were previously healthy, young, homosexual men living in Los Angeles. Soon, multiple similar reports surfaced as the illness we now recognize as AIDS revealed its ugly presence.

The AIDS story has been a catastrophic event in world history. An estimated thirty-seven million people worldwide currently live with AIDS, and over thirty-five million have died since its initial recognition in 1981. Fortunately, medicine has advanced dramatically over the past thirty-five years, and extended life expectancy is the norm. Unfortunately, despite these advances and the recent spending of over $20 billion for AIDS treatments, over nine hundred thousand people died of AIDS-related diseases worldwide in 2017. Just as concerning, there may be a slight upward trend in the incidence of this disease recently.

Remarkably, AIDS is essentially a preventable disease. Sexual abstinence, condoms, and some retroviral therapy used for infected individuals can reduce transmission by up to 100 percent if used properly. As with other diseases, however, commitment to prevention is frequently ignored by those most susceptible to this illness. And all the effort being used to treat and eliminate this disease has yet to consistently eradicate a severe medical issue that currently afflicts more than one million people in the United States.

AIDS, however, is not alone as a largely preventable illness.

Five Common Causes of Death

The five most common causes of death in the US are heart disease, cancer, stroke, lower respiratory diseases, and accidents (unintentional injuries). Besides valvular disease, the remaining four entities are largely preventable by optimizing certain risk factors. Cigarette use is the one preventable risk for four of the five leading causes of death. It is no wonder that both the government and the medical field labor tirelessly to eradicate this habit. Let us look at these common causes of death in more detail.

Heart disease:

Heart disease is a broad term that encompasses many illnesses, such as valvular disease, CAD, heart attacks, congestive heart failure, and rhythm abnormalities. While it also includes congenital heart disease and primary muscle disorders of the heart, these are much less common and rarely result in death. Heart disease can be prevented, as cigarette use, obesity, poor nutrition, diabetes, and inactivity are the main culprits. Reducing or eliminating these risk factors would substantially impact overall cardiovascular death rates in the US and worldwide.

Inactivity is also a largely avoidable risk. It's known that there's an inverse association between a person's cardiorespiratory fitness and the risk of cardiovascular death. In addition, the benefit of survival continues to extend as fitness improves, "with no upper limit." Recently, a Harvard-published study of male firefighters revealed that cardiovascular survival was markedly enhanced (96 percent reduction in cardiovascular events) in the group capable of performing forty or more push-ups compared to those unable to complete ten push-ups. This study further identifies overall fitness levels with cardiovascular risk and recognizes the importance of regular exercise as a preventative measure.

Cancer:

Cancer is used interchangeably with "malignancy" when discussing tumors and is the second most common cause of death. Over 1.7 million new cancer cases are diagnosed yearly in the United States. The most common is breast cancer, while the second most common (and deadliest) is lung cancer. Prostate cancer, colorectal malignancies, and melanoma round out the top five cancers in the US, and the top four malignancies in Europe mirror the US findings. Assessment of preventable risk factors in both Europe and the US has shown that five major lifestyle changes would dramatically reduce the burden of malignancies. Tobacco use remains the number one environmental cause of preventable diseases, while poor dietary habits, obesity, physical inactivity, and alcohol consumption are substantial risk factors for developing various malignancies.

High BMI is also linked to increased breast cancer risk, and the use of hormonal contraception may also increase risk, given the modest link between birth control use and breast cancer. Colorectal malignancies are associated with a high BMI and can be significantly reduced with increased vegetables and fruit in the diet. One can reduce melanoma risk by using appropriate sun protection and avoiding tanning beds.

Stroke:

Stroke risk is primarily related to blood pressure elevation, diabetes (up to four times increased risk of stroke), blood lipid abnormalities, and atrial fibrillation (irregular heart rhythm). Atrial fibrillation is associated with an increased risk of stroke in older patients (greater than age sixty-four) and those with a history of congestive heart failure, high blood pressure, diabetes, and other vascular abnormalities. Having experienced a previous neurologic event puts a patient at significant risk of recurrent stroke.

Since blood pressure is a risk factor, you want to optimize it through weight loss, some sodium restriction, and regular low-level exercise. An increased potassium intake and a healthier dietary regimen heavy on plants, including some fruits, and healthy fats are also advantageous. Reducing or eliminating alcohol in high-risk individuals may also have significant benefits, especially in those who engage in binge drinking.

Lower respiratory diseases:

Lower respiratory diseases affect up to thirty million people in the US and are most frequently linked to smoking. As previously stated, cigarette use is the single most significant health hazard related to poor health. Aggressive measures to lower risk have been met with limited success, but some promising results appear to be linked to the taxation of smoking products and restrictive laws regarding public smoking. Education seems to have some benefits based on reducing cigarette use in teenagers, but there has been an alarming rise (1,800 percent increase between 2011 and 2019) in teenage vaping. In addition, a recent study related to e-cigarette use showed that those who vape had a twofold increased risk of heart attack and an even greater risk of stroke. The fivefold greater risk for those who use cigarettes and e-cigarettes was of more significant concern. Vaping has also been associated with "popcorn lung," an insidious inflammatory lung disease that is particularly difficult to treat and is likely related to inhaled chemicals in the vaping material.

It remains unclear if marijuana use is linked to an increased risk of lung cancer. Few studies address this risk due to the illegality of marijuana in large segments of the country and patient recruitment and analysis limitations. In general, it would be reasonable to state that smoking any substance for any significant time is expected to be associated with an increased risk of pulmonary disease.

Accidents:

Motor vehicle accidents and accidental falls are the primary causes of unintentional injuries. A significant percentage of these injuries are largely preventable. In 2020, motorcyclists accounted for approximately 13 percent of all traffic fatalities, even though motorcycles comprise only 3 percent of registered vehicles on the road. Over 25 percent of motorcycle deaths were associated with alcohol use, and approximately 90 percent of the riders were male. In addition, 35 percent of those fatalities were riders aged 50 or above, with diminished reflex time and relative inexperience likely being contributing factors. Not surprisingly, helmet use was significantly effective in preventing death. This benefit of helmets extends to bicycle use as well.

Falls among the elderly are a huge problem. Some statistics suggest that the risk of death for those over sixty-five who fall and fracture their hip approaches 30 percent. This statistic is staggering when considering the opportunity for prevention among older individuals. Overall muscle mass begins to decline during our fourth decade of life. Although this process is inevitable, it can be altered positively with weight-bearing exercises. The advantage of walking, jogging, weightlifting, jumping rope, and other muscle-loading activities can significantly slow this loss of skeletal muscle. These activities are critically important as osteoporosis becomes more paramount among older individuals. Osteoporosis is not a disease that is exclusive to women.

Consequently, measures to enhance skeletal muscle strength and overall mass can significantly alter the magnitude of this issue in all people as they age. Flexibility and balance exercises are also critically important. One should begin as early in life as feasible, but it is never too late to start a weightlifting and aerobic exercise program. Sadly, weightlifting is one of the least favorite activities for most individuals, yet it can yield immense benefits on overall longevity and health. Therefore, I encourage all my patients to follow a twice weekly weightlifting program in addition to their aerobic exercise regimen. Adding one to two days of high-intensity interval training can also significantly blunt the loss of endurance and stabilize our body's capacity to extract oxygen during exercise (VO2 max). There is ample evidence to suggest that higher VO2 max levels are associated with improved overall health and lifespan. Therefore, moderate exercise is the most effective way to maintain good health and extend life.

Unintentional falls are also largely preventable with careful surveillance of home environment risks. Reviewing a patient's use of medications that may cause cognitive issues (antidepressants and sleep aids in particular) and medications that may cause low blood pressure can markedly diminish the risk of injury. And regular exercise and muscle strengthening can be highly effective tools to improve mobility in older individuals. One such exercise is dancing, which has the benefit of improving mobility and agility and has the added benefit of reducing the risk of dementia in the elderly.

Poison:

Prescription drug overdose is the leading cause of poisoning-related deaths, and opiate overdose has reached epidemic levels in the United States. Approximately 5 percent of pain medication abusers eventually use heroin, linked to a high risk of accidental overdose and death. The means of reducing and preventing this evolution is evident in the progressive restrictions on prescription medications, but criminal access and abuse remain significant issues. Fentanyl overdose in this country has also been an overwhelming cause of accidental death. Ongoing efforts to stem this rising tide of human devastation and loss have yet to achieve meaningful results.

Medical Errors:

One additional preventable cause of death is a topic that is perhaps not well-recognized and fully acknowledged by the medical community. A recent study by Johns Hopkins University brought attention to the alarming fact that medical errors rank as the third leading cause of death in the United States. The study highlighted many deaths resulting from incorrect diagnoses, inappropriate treatments, and medication errors. This emphasizes the crucial need for shared decision-making between doctors and patients, prioritizing careful consideration when prescribing medications and determining appropriate medical interventions.

It is crucial to note that this issue does not imply that doctors are untrustworthy or lacking competence. Instead, it reveals a systemic problem that likely stems from inconsistent levels of care and insufficient recognition of risks associated with medications and procedures.

Golden Prevention Rules

The most important and least difficult means to prevent illness and reduce all disease is to adhere to the five golden prevention rules: don't smoke, eat healthy, exercise, reduce stress, and sleep well.

There is no actual cost involved other than the money spent on good food and quality exercise equipment.

- Heart attacks and death can be reduced by 50 percent by eliminating cigarette use.
- Reducing low-quality sugars and processed foods in our diet can reduce inflammation and the harmful effects of insulin resistance.
- Exercise has multiple positive benefits on health and longevity, even in small incremental doses of ten to fifteen minutes a day.
- Stress reduction augments the survival curve for cardiac events in a significant manner.
- Sleep duration of six to nine hours each night is strongly linked to longevity and a decline in common illnesses.

Most individuals desire a long life to savor their retirement, enjoy their grandchildren, and "see the world." Sadly, many of my patients do not achieve their dreams because of poor health. I often hear that the golden years are spent in doctors' offices, pharmacies, and hospitals.

As an interventional cardiologist, I freely admit the incredible satisfaction and "rush" that I felt when I could open an acutely occluded coronary artery of a heart attack patient and almost instantaneously change the course of their life. However, I did not want to be the medical firefighter who had to rush into the hospital to extinguish the acute flame of injury inside someone's chest. I have always felt a duty and a calling to be the fire safety officer who screens each patient's risks and hazards to avoid health catastrophes before they arrive.

We must change our approach to health and recognize that prevention is the pathway to cure. Medicine and health are not that complex. Treatment is simple if we can develop good habits and cast-off bad choices. Do not be discouraged. The biblical quote "take up his mat and walk" comes from the story of Jesus healing a man who had been paralyzed for thirty-eight years. When Jesus saw the man lying by the pool, he asked him if he wanted to be healed. The man replied that he had no one to help him into the pool when the water was stirred, which was believed to have healing properties. Jesus then commanded the man to "get up, pick up your mat, and walk" (John 5:8).

In the same way, adopting a healthy lifestyle can help us to "take up our mat and walk" toward a better life. When we make healthy choices, such as eating a balanced diet, exercising regularly, getting enough sleep, and reducing stress, we can experience numerous benefits. We can have more energy, feel physically and mentally better, and reduce our risk of developing chronic diseases such as heart disease, diabetes, and cancer.

Just as Jesus commanded the paralyzed man to act and take control of his life, we, too, can make positive changes in our lives. A healthy lifestyle can improve our overall well-being and help us enjoy a better quality of life. So, let us take our mats and walk toward a healthier and happier life. Good health awaits you, but it takes hard work in the beginning. As physicians, many of us promise to be with you every step of the way.

I remind you of one of my favorite medical quotes as you journey onward:

"Medicine [is] the only profession that labors incessantly to destroy the reason for its existence."

James Bryce

Takeaways

1. Heart disease, cancer, stroke, lower respiratory diseases, and accidents (unintentional injuries) are the most common causes of death in the US.
2. A significant number of these deaths are preventable with appropriate measures.
3. Cigarette cessation is far and away the most effective way to prevent death and chronic disease.
4. Poor dietary habits, obesity, lack of exercise, and alcohol consumption lead to significant health deterioration and are largely avoidable with lifestyle changes.
5. Simple measures such as helmet use can mitigate the risk of traumatic brain injury.
6. Unintentional falls in older populations are an unrecognized cause of premature death.

Chapter 7

Supplements

"My mother made us eat all sorts of vitamins and supplements until one day I nearly choked on part of The Sunday Times."

Milton Jones, comedian

Before the beginning of the twentieth century, many healthcare providers adhered to a homeopathic healthcare approach that focused on the benefits of nutrition and sanitation. Drug therapy was limited by a lack of supply, but available herbs and vitamin sources served as vital therapeutics for the care of the healthy and the ill. The "terrain theory" adhered to the premise that disease occurred primarily due to poor lifestyle, poor sanitation, nutritional deficiencies, and the absence of clean water. This integrative approach assumed that "germs" were a secondary factor that only caused disease when the health conditions were poor and had altered the underlying "terrain" in such a way as to allow unhealthy tissue to become infected. Many of the deadliest infectious diseases during this time were primarily spread through unsanitary living conditions or water contamination. Poor nutrition also played a role in making the body more susceptible to disease.

We still see this dynamic in many low-income countries today, where poverty leads to poor food sourcing, inadequate sanitation, and a lack of clean water. The consequences of these conditions are reflected in the mortality statistics of these countries, where the leading cause of death is lower respiratory infections and diarrheal diseases. Five of the top ten causes of death in impoverished countries are infectious. Although it is thought that vaccines and various medications have played a vital role in ameliorating these diseases, the historical data implies that mortality from most infectious diseases, including polio, was declining long before vaccines and antibiotics were available. The pasteurization of dairy products, improved sanitation, and open-water filtration systems have been the principal factors in eliminating these diseases and improving survival.

The "germ theory" was introduced in the late nineteenth century and espoused the premise that most human diseases result from different germs that enter the body and cause illness. Bacteria and viruses were the culprits and eliminating them became the primary target of the healthcare field. Vaccines and pharmaceutical agents were subsequently developed to wage war against these transmitters of disease.

Despite focusing on eliminating harmful bacteria and viruses through vaccines and pharmaceutical agents, the theory also highlighted the presence of beneficial bacteria and viruses in the human body. We now understand that many beneficial bacteria and viruses have evolved and existed, within and on the body's surface, which are essential to overall health. Gut bacteria are an excellent example of existing bacteria vital to human health. This knowledge has led to a deeper understanding of the essential role that healthy gut bacteria play in maintaining overall health and well-being. These organisms have what is known as a commensal relationship with our bodies. In other words, the existing bacteria in our body benefits us, and we benefit from the bacteria.

By recognizing the importance of these microorganisms, medical professionals can work to promote a healthy balance of bacteria and viruses within the body, which can lead to better health outcomes for individuals. Therefore, the germ theory has ultimately contributed to a more comprehensive approach to healthcare that recognizes the positive aspects of microorganisms in addition to their potential negative effects.

With that said, the germ theory also brought some drawbacks. Sadly, homeopathic treatments, natural therapeutics, nutritious foods, and herbs rich in vitamins and other beneficial qualities were abandoned or discouraged as the germ theory took a foothold in society. Physicians were heavily educated on this approach to medical care, and they became inundated with new drugs and vaccines as the primary treatment options for disease.

The broad use of antibiotics for all infections remains a mainstay of clinical practice today, even though widespread resistance to these agents continues. In addition, many upper respiratory and gastrointestinal infections are caused by viruses and do not respond to antibiotic treatment. Despite this, patients demand, and doctors usually comply with, more and more antibiotics. This drug-centered approach has extended dramatically into the field of cardiology during my career, and statin drugs and blood pressure medicines are some of the most prescribed and profit-producing medications today.

This drug-centered approach inspired by germ theory has resulted in dismissing or ignoring alternative treatment options and an emphasis on lifestyle changes. Nutrition instruction in medical school training is essentially nonexistent. Most physicians spend little time advancing the terrain theory in their practices.

Combining these two theories can lead to a more integrated approach to healthcare delivery. By recognizing the role of microorganisms in causing disease, healthcare professionals can focus on preventative measures such as vaccination and hygiene to limit exposure to harmful pathogens. However, they can also incorporate the terrain theory by addressing the underlying factors that affect the body's internal environment, such as diet, exercise, and stress management.

By combining these two theories, healthcare professionals can work to improve overall health outcomes for patients. This approach can lead to a more comprehensive and effective healthcare delivery system that addresses the root causes of illness and promotes long-term health and well-being.

I sincerely hope that a symbiotic relationship can develop that mixes the terrain and germ theories in the future delivery of healthcare. Patients will be the logical beneficiaries of this approach.

Nutritional Supplements Battle

As medical information becomes more easily accessible to the public, there is a growing interest in using nutritional supplements to maintain health. This counterbalance to the prevailing approach to medical care is quite refreshing and should be broadly welcomed by healthcare workers; however, there is an ongoing debate about the need for and overall effects of these products. A quiet battle continues between the established medical community and the rising tide of integrative healthcare providers. More healthcare providers are becoming interested in the integrative approach, and a small but influential group of integrative organizations are providing training for practicing physicians who want to learn more about an integrative approach. It is a tiny segment of the medical profession, especially within cardiology.

The pharmaceutical industry is also actively engaged in this debate, and one could logically assume that it is because any alternative to standard drug therapy negatively impacts its profitability. However, some evidence suggests that the pharmaceutical industry does have a significant influence on the healthcare field, which can impact the way that supplements are viewed and studied within the medical community.

One study published in the Cochrane Library found that industry funding was associated with higher rates of favorable results for drug and medical device studies. The study analyzed seventy-five drug and device trials published in several major medical journals between 2010 and 2015 and found that industry-funded trials were more likely to report positive results than trials that were not industry funded. This suggests that industry funding can bias the results of medical research and may impact how specific treatments, including supplements, are viewed within the medical community. While it is essential to be cautious when interpreting these findings and not make broad generalizations about the medical research field, they do suggest that some bias exists in how supplements are viewed and studied within the medical community.

It's also worth noting that there is still an ongoing debate among healthcare professionals and researchers about the efficacy and safety of many supplements, and more research is needed to fully understand the potential benefits and risks associated with these products. At present, however, it seems unlikely that unbiased studies on nutritional supplement benefits will be published given the heavy influence of the pharmaceutical industry on the healthcare field. This is mainly reflected in major medical journals that have perceived conflicts of interest due to the financial support that they receive from the pharmaceutical industry.

Consequently, the battlefield is entirely blurred by the impact that economics and pseudoscience bring to bear. Prominent researchers and lead authors frequently have conflicts of interest related to receiving pharmaceutical companies' payments and salaries. As a result of this misdirection, allopathic physicians (MDs) such as myself have been slow to embrace and quick to criticize the use of alternative treatments in the care of patients. To their credit,

osteopathic physicians (DOs), chiropractors, and naturopathic practitioners have utilized these various treatments for an extended period. The internet now helps patients be more aware of these alternatives than at any other time in modern medical history.
It behooves all medical providers to at least educate themselves on the available information regarding supplements. Vitamins, herbs, and naturally occurring therapeutics are readily available for use in health and disease.

Valuable Supplements

Over time, I have tried to critically assess the value of some supplements. I have listed those agents that I believe have some intrinsic health benefits. I include only a limited number of them, but they are also essential supplements in my practice. I fully accept any criticism of my choices, but I invite skeptics to conduct thorough, unbiased investigations. I would also remind my readers that one can never out-supplement a lousy diet or a poor lifestyle. I also recommend that you always check for the potency of the supplements before purchase. Buying the cheapest product assuming all have the same efficacy, can be a significant error. Purity is also paramount. Blindly purchasing products at grocery stores or online websites without assurance of their quality can also be problematic and costly if the supplements are poorly made or have low potency.

My interest in supplements focuses on two main themes: inflammation reduction and immune enhancement. As my insight into patient care has evolved and changed, the following discussion will focus only on a limited number of available choices related to cardiovascular health. I genuinely believe that the following agents are advantageous for most individuals. That said, I leave it to the reader to do your own research to decide if any or all of these products may benefit your health journey. I must also emphasize the importance of obtaining the clearance and approval of your healthcare provider before starting any of these supplements. Some supplements may interact with your current medications. In addition, some supplements may not be safe in certain medical conditions. An example of this is the use of fish oil in patients who are on certain blood thinners, where an increase in bleeding risk may ensue.

Fish oil:

Fish oil has several advantages for the cardiovascular system. Multiple studies have revealed its benefits, mainly due to its anti-inflammatory effects from its components suppressing some pro-inflammatory substances. It contains DHA (docosahexaenoic acid) and EPA (eicosapentaenoic acid), two crucial free fatty acids that appear to benefit cardiovascular disease. When adequate doses are consumed, there is a reduction in triglycerides and an increase in good cholesterol (HDL). It also has a beneficial effect on the brain—an enhancement in memory and a reduction in cognitive decline has been reported, as well as a reduction in depression. Given its anti-inflammatory qualities, it is not surprising that fish oil may also have therapeutic effects on asthma, skin diseases, and arthritis symptoms. Krill oil may have similar or more significant advantages and better absorption than regular fish oil.

For those who are interested, there is an available assay (omega-3 index) that identifies if the appropriate amount of fish oil is being consumed to benefit overall health. Taking a total daily dose of 2.0–2.5 grams of combined DHA and EPA for efficacy is essential. Remember that fish oil products also contain both vitamins A and D. As a reminder, patients on non-aspirin blood thinners should avoid fish oil supplements to avoid the potential enhanced bleeding risk. However, these patients can still obtain omega-3 fatty acids from modest weekly fish consumption.

Magnesium:

While magnesium is number twelve on the periodic table, it should be close to the top of the list of important elements in our body. It is essential for the activity of nearly six hundred biological enzymes and is required to produce energy. In the US, we have a real issue with magnesium deficiency, which is likely related to decreased consumption of high-magnesium-containing foods (green vegetables, nuts, avocado) and diminished absorption from the gut and kidney (often related to inflammatory bowel disease, diarrhea, and kidney disease). Furthermore, over the past few decades, the amount of available magnesium in foods has decreased by 30–40 percent due to several factors, including soil depletion and farming techniques.

Certain common drugs (such as proton pump inhibitors for treating esophageal and gastric issues) block magnesium absorption. Diuretics, oral contraceptives, chronic alcohol use, and diabetes can all contribute to low magnesium levels. Low magnesium levels have been strongly linked to diabetes risk, cardiovascular diseases (including atherosclerosis and heart arrhythmias), osteoporosis, hypertension, depression, and many other conditions. In my experience, atrial fibrillation's incidence has exploded, as verified in the literature. I have often wondered if magnesium deficiency significantly affects this incidence. Supplementation can have significant advantages in treating these various maladies.

One important caveat is that the typical blood test for magnesium levels measures only about 1 percent of the total body magnesium and can be very misleading. Sixty percent of magnesium is stored in bone and cannot be accurately measured in a blood test.

Men need at least 400–500 mg of elemental magnesium daily, while women need 300–400 mg daily. Increased magnesium loss from sweating or bowel-related issues will require more replenishment. Individuals who use drugs such as diuretics or proton pump inhibitors must also adjust their intake. It is essential to clarify that bioavailable magnesium varies widely among supplements. Adequate absorption from the GI tract makes magnesium oxide and citrate less reliable. I generally use magnesium malate and glycinate for most of my patients. Magnesium threonate is also very beneficial for sleep-related issues because it more readily crosses the blood-brain barrier.

CoQ10:

CoQ10, also known as ubiquinone and its active form ubiquinol, is a natural, "ubiquitous" substance present in every cell of the body, best known for its antioxidant features. It has a dualistic role, playing an integral part in energy production and serving as an antioxidant to neutralize the free radicals generated in that process. CoQ10 is found in the highest concentrations in organs that produce the most energy (heart, liver, kidneys, and brain). It diminishes as we age and is further reduced by certain drugs such as statins, beta-blockers, tricyclic antidepressants, and some diabetes medications, including metformin. As a result, supplementing this substance can help lower the risk of free radical damage that would otherwise lead to cell breakdown and death.

A Swedish study showed the benefits of CoQ10 and selenium in a randomized clinical trial that involved 443 healthy elderly participants who received either 200 mg of CoQ10 and 200 mcg of selenium daily or a placebo for four years. The study aimed to evaluate the effects of the supplements on cardiovascular mortality and morbidity, as well as on oxidative stress and inflammation.

They found that the supplementation group had:

- a 49 percent lower heart-related death rate than the placebo group after four years of intervention and twelve years of follow-up

- a lower rate of hospitalization due to heart failure and a better cardiac function as measured by echocardiography
- lower levels of biomarkers of oxidative stress and inflammation than the placebo group
- higher levels of selenium and CoQ10 in plasma than the placebo group, indicating good compliance and bioavailability of the supplements

The study concluded that CoQ10 and selenium supplementation in elderly individuals with low selenium status can have long-lasting beneficial effects on cardiovascular health and survival, as well as on oxidative stress and inflammation. The study also suggested that CoQ10 and selenium may have synergistic effects on cellular energy production and antioxidant defense.

Inadequate CoQ10 has also been linked to some neurodegenerative diseases, such as Parkinson's disease and possibly ALS, and it may also be associated with cognitive dysfunction and decline. Low levels of CoQ10 have also been associated with cardiac dysfunction, muscle soreness, and weakness in statin users. I always supplement statin therapy with CoQ10 because of the high incidence of these symptoms in my patient population. CoQ10 is also effective for hypertension and some forms of congestive heart failure. Of most significant importance, however, are its antioxidant benefits and positive effect on cellular longevity. There are some side effects of CoQ10, but doses of even more than 1200 mg daily can be ingested with relative safety if approved by a qualified healthcare expert.

Essential vitamins:

Essential vitamins are those vitamins that our body requires but cannot produce in the amount that is necessary for survival. The essential vitamins include A, B, C, D, E, and K. There are eight different B vitamins.

Vitamin D3. Vitamin D and vitamin D3 are not the same. Vitamin D is a general term for a group of fat-soluble vitamins important for many body functions. There are two main forms of vitamin D: vitamin D2 (ergocalciferol) and vitamin D3 (cholecalciferol). Vitamin D2 comes from plants and fortified foods, while vitamin D3 primarily comes from sunlight exposure. Vitamin D3 is more potent and effective than vitamin D2 in raising and maintaining the blood levels of vitamin D, which is essential for bone health, immune function, and other benefits. Therefore, vitamin D3 is the preferred form of vitamin D for supplementation. As a result, sun exposure plays a role in its production, but it must be converted to its active form by the liver and the kidney. Vitamin D receptors (VDRs) have been discovered throughout the body, revealing that vitamin D activity is broad. While this vitamin is known mainly for its impact on calcium absorption and bone integrity, it also plays a role in immunity. It appears to positively impact cellular and vascular inflammation. Some studies show a positive link between obesity and vitamin D deficiency; vitamin D3 replenishment may reduce the risk of type 2 diabetes.

Additionally, vitamin D3 supplements appear to lower blood pressure in some patients. In cardiovascular terms, a deficiency of vitamin D3 has been linked to an increased risk of stroke and resistant hypertension, impacting overall survival. There also is evidence that vitamin D3 deficiency is linked to cognitive dysfunction and possible Alzheimer's risk. One recent study revealed that vitamin D deficiency in older patients is linked to a significant reduction in long-term muscle strength.

One additional benefit of vitamin D supplementation is related to its impact on cancer. The recent DO-HEALTH study revealed that patients who used a combination of vitamin D supplementation with fish oil and weekly strength training had a 61 percent reduction in invasive cancer risk. This impact is substantial.

It should be mentioned that the science is not settled about vitamin D supplementation. My approach is hopefully pragmatic.

Given the extensive role that vitamin D3 plays in many critical biologic processes and the negative impacts of vitamin D deficiency, it seems appropriate to consider some vitamin D supplementation for at-risk individuals. Vitamin D3 levels are easily measured and can guide treatment. I suggest 5000 units of vitamin D3 daily for most adults, but kidney or liver disease or other health issues would alter this amount. Patients must always check with their medical provider before indiscriminately taking any supplements.

Vitamin C. Vitamin C is classified as an essential vitamin. Vitamin C is an integral player in many biochemical processes in the body, primarily serving as an antioxidant and free radical scavenger to reduce oxidative damage at the cellular and vascular levels. There is some imbalance in the scientific literature regarding this vital vitamin. Still, it appears that vitamin C taken in doses of at least 500 mg/day has a beneficial role in cardiovascular disease and possibly cancers. This makes sense when considering the positive effect of antioxidants in reducing inflammation. Regular supplementation of vitamin C is associated with a relative risk reduction (greater than 25 percent) of cardiovascular events and stroke. This value is similar to the results of statin drugs but without the attendant side effects. Vitamin C also appears to have a beneficial impact on cholesterol levels and blood pressure.

Vitamin K. K vitamins are a group of fat-soluble vitamins that play an essential role in blood clotting and bone health.

There are two main types of vitamin K: K1 (phylloquinone) and K2 (menaquinone). K1 is primarily found in leafy greens and is essential for blood clotting, while K2 comes in several forms, including K2-MK4 and K2-MK7.

K2-MK4 is found in animal products, such as meat, egg yolks, and dairy, and is essential for bone health. K2-MK7, on the other hand, is produced by bacteria and is found in fermented foods like natto and cheese.

Both forms of K2 play a role in directing calcium to the bones and teeth and away from soft tissues like arteries, which can help prevent calcification and improve cardiovascular health. The K2 vitamins play an important role in cardiovascular health. K2-MK4 and K2-MK7 activate a decalcification protein that ultimately lessens calcification of the arterial wall and may also lessen arterial stiffness. Arterial stiffness is associated with higher blood pressure risk, and calcification of the coronary arteries is linked to higher overall cardiac events such as heart attacks and cardiovascular death.

One intriguing possible benefit of vitamin MK4/MK7 supplementation is related to statin therapy and its known effect of increasing coronary calcification. Statins are thought to stabilize soft, unstable cholesterol plaques in the arteries and make them more calcified and stable, perhaps because of the anti-inflammatory activity of these drugs. Interestingly, however, statins also block the synthesis of vitamin K2, which is essential to preventing arterial calcification. For this reason, I believe that MK4/MK7 supplementation can benefit patients who are taking statin therapy. This supplement regimen may be even more important in those patients who do not have an adequate intake of green vegetables in their diet.

I also offer the option of vitamin MK4/MK7 supplementation for my patients with calcific aortic and mitral valve disease. The current medical treatment to slow the progress of aortic and mitral stenosis is very limited. Adding MK4/MK7 in conjunction with vitamin D3 as an attempt to slow or reverse the calcification process of the tissue valve makes sense based on the scientific evidence. I give this option to all my patients who have these cardiac issues. In my limited observational experience, some patients seem to have stabilization of their aortic stenosis when they consistently take this combination therapy. I hope that future studies will clarify if this regimen improves their progress and lowers the need for surgical intervention. Only time will tell.

Many people in the US have a vitamin K deficiency. Still, it is unclear if this plays a vital role in the overall higher incidence of cardiovascular disease. In laboratory studies, supplementation with

MK4/MK7 has been shown to reduce arterial calcification. A large observational study also linked increased dietary K2 intake to reducing cardiovascular mortality. My approach is to supplement with MK4/MK7 in combination with vitamin D3 to enhance the activation of osteocalcin (for bone growth) and reduce arterial and tissue calcification. I generally use between 100–320 mg daily, but I favor the higher dose to offset any reduction in dietary vitamin K intake that might be present in individual patients. Although vitamin K is the source of vitamin K2 availability, it is difficult for many patients to get adequate amounts of bioavailable vitamin K2 through diet alone.

Recent research has revealed that vitamin K2 may have significant benefits unrelated to its cardiovascular effects. Vitamin K also plays a role in activating osteocalcin, a substance that inhibits the calcification of soft tissues, appears to facilitate bone growth, and plays a role in glucose control. It has also been associated with enhanced bone growth, diminished tissue calcification, and reduced diabetes risk.

It appears to have antioxidant features and may reduce the incidence of cancer and diabetes. One large study revealed a 7 percent reduction in diabetes risk with vitamin K2 supplementation of just 10 mg daily.

Before starting this supplement, individuals on warfarin and other blood thinners must seek counsel and obtain clearance from their medical providers. This is exceptionally important. Those with chronic kidney disease appear at high risk for vitamin K1 and K2 deficiency and are known to have an enhanced risk of arterial and heart valve calcification. This group may benefit from this supplement as long as they are not on concurrent blood thinners.

Quercetin:

Quercetin is a plant chemical found in the pigment of certain foods, including various fruits, legumes (beans, peas, peanuts), tea, and dark chocolate. It is known for its antioxidant and anti-inflammatory capabilities and helps reduce cellular damage. Furthermore, quercetin has been used to diminish viral-induced cellular inflammatory reactions and appears to enhance immunity. I have used quercetin (500 mg once or twice daily) in combination with vitamin D3 (5000 units daily), zinc picolinate (11–50 mg daily), and vitamin C (500 mg twice daily) for improved immunity during the COVID-19 pandemic. By combining this regimen with a whole food diet that is highly plant-based, regular exercise, calorie restriction, and good sleep habits, I feel that individuals can take a proactive role in reducing the risk of COVID-19 and other viral infections. In addition, using natural and easily obtainable anti-inflammatory agents can also undercut the cause of many different inflammatory conditions such as CAD, hypertension, insulin resistance, diabetes, and chronic joint disorders. There is also some interesting evidence that quercetin may diminish the risk of cognitive decline and Alzheimer's disease.

Side effects are infrequent, and it makes common sense to me to strongly encourage an increased intake of this valuable nutrient.

Although many believe that wine is rich in polyphenols, the total concentration is relatively small. Red wine has the highest flavonoid concentration, especially Syrah or Shiraz.

Plums are also very high in flavonoid concentration but are not always in season. Berries (especially acai berries, blueberries, and raspberries) are a plentiful and tasty source of these beneficial antioxidants. Dried parsley, Mexican dried oregano, and cacao beans have some of the highest flavonoids, and it would be wise to incorporate these nutrients into your diet.

Turmeric:

Turmeric is a spice that originates from a root in the ginger family. It appears to have antioxidant, anti-inflammatory, and antitumor qualities. Although much focus has been placed on the active substance in turmeric—called curcumin—there seem to be additional health-giving benefits in many of the other breakdown products of this root. These "curcuminoids" play a role in the GI tract and may positively alter the gut bacteria to reduce intestinal inflammation. This effect may beneficially alter the gut-brain axis and protect the brain. The gut-brain axis is a two-way communication pathway between the digestive system (the gut) and the central nervous system (the brain). Various hormonal, immune, and neural pathways facilitate this communication. The gut-brain axis regulates many bodily functions, including digestion, mood, and immune function. Most chronic adult diseases appear to occur because of underlying inflammation; logically, foods and spices that reduce inflammation will benefit people with these diseases.

Turmeric appears to be especially beneficial in diabetes management and slowing cognitive decline. It may play a valuable role in cancer prevention based on its ability to reduce blood vessel growth in and enhance the programmed death of tumor cells.

A recent meta-analysis of several trials related to cholesterol and turmeric revealed a significantly positive benefit of turmeric extracts on LDL and triglyceride levels in patients, with few to no side effects at even higher doses.

Although the absorption of turmeric and curcumin can be pretty variable based on the commercial product, as little as 250 mg of oral curcumin daily has been shown to reduce insulin resistance and diminish the progression of type 2 diabetes. There is also clinical evidence of its beneficial effects on inflammatory joint conditions. It has long been used for its therapeutic effect on certain inflammatory gastrointestinal diseases. All in all, the myriad benefits of this widely available food product make it a perfect choice for daily use in meals and drinks. As more studies evaluate the role of bioavailable curcumin extracts, we should expect an even more significant benefit from this beautiful "golden spice."

Glucosamine:

One other supplement that has gained my attention is glucosamine. This amino sugar is commonly used to relieve joint inflammation and arthritis symptoms. Glucosamine sulfate at a dose of 500 mg three times daily has been shown to have some therapeutic benefits in some people by providing nutrient support to the cartilage in our bone structure. Of greater importance, however, is pretty strong evidence that glucosamine supplementation positively impacts all-cause mortality (15 percent reduction), cardiovascular mortality (18 percent reduction), and cancer and respiratory mortality. The causes and effects remain unclear, but glucosamine possesses anti-inflammatory properties that are beneficial in reducing multiple chronic disease states such as cardiovascular disease and diabetes.

Citrus Bergamot:

Citrus bergamot is a unique fruit that is found in the southern part of Italy and is high in beneficial phytochemicals. Bergamot appears to have many benefits that are related to its unique antioxidant and anti-inflammatory effects. It has been shown to diminish blood pressure and blood glucose in some studies but its greatest benefit may be related to its favorable effects on lipids. Several studies have revealed that Bergamot at doses of 500 mg-1000 mg daily reduced total cholesterol, LDL cholesterol and triglyceride levels. In addition, HDL levels improved. One important study revealed that this valuable fruit also changed the size of the LDL particles from the more dangerous small dense LDL to the larger and less harmful LDL.

Treating COVID-19 with Supplements

One final word seems necessary when considering COVID-19 and other viral illnesses. Almost all government emphasis on treatment has focused on vaccines and therapeutics such as remdesivir and monoclonal antibodies. There has been a "deafening silence" from the COVID-19 task force members regarding the importance of a healthy lifestyle and alternative treatments such as targeted nutrients. This has been maddening for many of us who currently treat this illness.

On a positive note, Pfizer and Merck have recently created specific oral antiviral drug therapies. Pfizer has reported 90 percent efficacy for its pill in reducing hospitalization and death if it is taken early in the infection. If these early indicators are accurate, this would rival the vaccine results and may well supplant the continuing need for booster therapy. Sadly, however, the near-complete absence of advice promoting enhanced immunity is lost in this intense search for effective treatment.

I often liken disease treatment to a football game: you need a good offense (drugs and other medical treatments) and a good defense (healthy lifestyle and targeted supplements). As to COVID-19 treatment, we have the medicines and vaccines, yet we continue to see large numbers of infections even in vaccinated patients. After caring for many hospitalized COVID-19 patients, I am convinced that optimizing good eating habits, exercising regularly, and getting optimum sleep is crucial in the war to reduce risk. In addition, targeted supplements may have a role. I include the following combination as an immune "package" for my patients worried about viral exposure to COVID-19 and possibly other viral infections such as influenza. Since COVID-19 will likely not be going away, it is reasonable for some to use this daily regimen. Patients should always check with their healthcare provider before starting this regimen.

- Vitamin C: 500–1000 mg twice daily
- Quercetin: 250–500 mg daily
- Vitamin D: 4000–7000 units daily (higher amounts for higher BMI)
- Elemental zinc: 15–30 mg daily (100 mg of zinc picolinate will provide 20 mg of essential zinc. Be aware of the interaction of copper and excess zinc consumption. High zinc levels can limit copper absorption. Increasing dietary intake of copper [oysters, salmon, dark chocolate, nuts, shitake mushrooms, avocado, and sweet potato] can offset this risk.)

Over the next few years, COVID-19 will likely continue to be a serious player in the healthcare field. As potential patients, all of us should become well prepared by enhancing our immunity so we will become less susceptible to the ravages of this troublesome disease.

Daily Supplement Regimen

It is difficult to give one specific regimen because everyone has different eating patterns, activities, and sun exposure experiences. In addition, drug interactions may be a factor. For this reason, I again remind each person that checking with your healthcare provider is essential before starting any supplement regimen.

With that said, you can consider the following:

- Fish oil: 2000–3000 mg daily
- Vitamin D3: 5000iu daily
- Vitamin K2/K7: 90–120 ug daily
- Magnesium: 400–800 mg daily (I prefer glycinate or malate)

- Glucosamine sulfate: 1500 mg total per day in divided doses (750 mg twice daily)
- Quercetin: 500 mg one to two times daily
- CoQ10: 100–200 mg daily (I prefer oil or lipid based for better absorption
- Vitamin C: 500 mg twice daily
- Turmeric: 500–1000 mg daily

This is an incomplete list for some people, but many supplements benefit brain and vascular health and immune support. I would also remind everyone that the ideal source of these nutrients would be healthy, nutrient-dense foods. Still, achieving the optimum levels with limited dietary consumption alone can be difficult. I would also again emphasize that no number of supplements can overcome the health consequences of a bad diet or inadequate exercise and sleep. We should not adhere to the false premise that herbs and vitamins will supplant the need for good lifestyle habits. Identifying and monitoring for any unusual side effects is also critically important. Always be honest with your healthcare provider when initiating any new supplement.

__Takeaways__

1. Modern medical care has focused on the germ theory with an overemphasis on medications. The terrain theory offers a better integrative approach to overall health by focusing on a healthy lifestyle, clean water, sanitation infrastructure, and targeted nutritional supplementation to enhance health and immunity.
2. Quality supplements are essential due to potential potency and toxicity issues that can cause harm and ineffectiveness.
3. ALWAYS check with your primary care provider regarding supplementation and weigh the risks versus benefits when

instituting targeted therapy.
4. Fish oil, vitamin D3, vitamin C, and vitamin K2/K7 are likely beneficial for most individuals focused on brain and cardiovascular health. K2/K7 should be avoided in those individuals with clotting disorders or who are taking blood thinners.
5. Magnesium plays a vital role in many biochemical processes and is an effective tool for blood pressure and sleep. Most individuals have some degree of magnesium deficiency.
6. Targeted supplementation with quercetin, vitamin D3, vitamin C, and zinc may reduce the risk of some viral illnesses, including COVID-19.

Chapter 8

Spirituality

"Diseases of the soul are more dangerous and more numerous than those of the body."

Marcus Tullius Cicero

I approach this topic of spirituality from a Judeo-Christian perspective, but I believe any religion that ascribes to a loving and caring God or the divine can understand my beliefs.

It is incredible how much of our personal development is experiential. Our interactions with our environment and the individuals who influence our life directly impact what we value and how we approach others. In addition, our parents, spouses, teachers, and friends often play vital roles in shaping our personalities and opinions.

My wife is one of my strongest inspirations. Many years ago, she played a formative role in my recognition of spiritual engagement and prayer as a vital medical care component. She had discovered a small breast lump that we both thought was insignificant. Nevertheless, she wanted to be diligent in her evaluation because we had two young children to nurture. The breast surgeon performed a needle biopsy, revealing a rare malignancy that affects both breasts frequently. The news turned our world upside down. My courageous and profoundly spiritual wife faced this news with great determination and asked me to begin a prayer group before her surgery.

The outpouring of love and support was immediate, and we were overwhelmed by the number of individuals who started to pray for her. Before her surgery, I went running to dissipate some of my anxiety and worry. Along the way, I found a worn Bible lying along the road and brought it home. When I showed my wife this discovery, an immediate peace came upon her. Intuitively, she knew that all would now be well. Later that evening, I received the news from my two surgical friends in the recovery room that the tumor was inexplicably benign, and no further treatment was necessary. Prayers had been answered. The intense emotion of that moment remains vivid and influential to this day. It has motivated me and convinced me that prayer is a vital and integral component of treatment and healing. Nothing will convince me otherwise.

As physicians, personal interactions with patients can be a unique opportunity to promote a culture of spirituality and true holiness. At its core, spirituality involves the pursuit of a deeper relationship with God or a divine entity. This relationship is based on faith, trust, and a desire to connect with the divine presence in a meaningful way. Whether it involves prayer, meditation, the study of religious texts, or acts of service and kindness, spirituality is a means of deepening one's relationship with God and aligning oneself with divine will. This relationship is personal and intimate, and it provides a sense of comfort, guidance, and purpose in life. Regardless of the specific religious tradition, the pursuit of a deeper relationship with God or the divine is a central aspect of spirituality and a means of finding meaning and fulfillment in life.

Some may take offense to this statement, but every physician could introduce the three theological virtues of faith, hope, and love during personal patient interactions. For the agnostic or nonbeliever, these virtues can be viewed as universal altruistic qualities allowing our patients to trust our capabilities and knowledge (faith). It can offer them encouragement to recover or heal (hope). It also teaches them that we are present and compassionate providers who genuinely care for their health and well-being (love). Doctors are often criticized for our arrogance and our inability to listen genuinely. Instilling a spiritual component to patient care can nurture both the patient and the physician. Physicians can also serve as a personal support system for patients struggling with interpersonal or ongoing medical issues that would benefit from the injection of faith and hope. I know that it has been an invaluable addition to my patient interactions.

In medical school, we had abundant required reading and an extensive curriculum to fulfill course requirements. The focus was on the scientific method of disease and healing. Much of this process was tedious and perhaps unnecessary to the application of my future practice of clinical medicine. Noticeably absent was any substantive requirement regarding the humanities and the interrelationship between science and reason. Spirituality was primarily ignored, even though abundant research has revealed spirituality's vital role in health and disease. Even though I attended a medical school founded on a Catholic tradition, exposure to Christian ideals such as prayer, meditation, and emphasis on developing a personal relationship with God was left mainly to the individual. Only limited guidance was provided to incorporate a humanistic approach into our medical training.

Ultimately, the question of spirituality and religious engagement must be analyzed scientifically, and this is where the crossroads of science and observational bias frequently collide. In my extensive review of the literature, there appears to be a remarkably positive correlation between cardiovascular disease outcomes and religious engagement. Unfortunately, the medical community's response to these studies has ranged from skepticism to outright condemnation. To some extent, this is understandable.

After all, the Semmelweis reflex is a human behavioral tendency to reject new information or knowledge that contradicts established beliefs or norms. The scientific community and the medical field have struggled to accept spirituality as a causative factor in health outcomes. This attitude assumes that science is pure and unbiased, yet this is not true. We frequently see manipulation of scientific data to support results and biases in the media and medical journals. In my experience, the adverse reaction to medical studies that reveal the benefits of spiritual interventions seems more robust and dismissive within the medical community. The media and the lay community then criticize or ignore such studies on the pretense that the narrative is not in unity with the prevailing theories regarding health and disease. This may explain why physicians avoid discussing spirituality in their offices or hospital settings.

But over my medical career, I have realized that humanity's physical and spiritual essence is inseparable, mainly when dealing with health and disease. I have often reminded my patients that as human beings, our existence embodies both physical and spiritual elements. Yet many of us spend lavish amounts of time and money on our physical component but neglect or completely ignore the spiritual part. As a Christian physician, I lament this realization. It is a collective tragedy that we fail to recognize the value of incorporating a spiritual component into the spectrum of human health and disease.

Relationship between Spirituality and Health

Historically, physicians have interlaced spirituality and healing since the third century. Many of the early physicians were also priests in their culture. The twin physicians Cosmas and Damian attended to their patients' physical and spiritual needs in the fourth century and are recognized as saints in the Catholic Church. They were known as the Holy Unmercenaries, a devoted group of physicians throughout history who served patients' spiritual and medical needs without any payment.

Prayer, fasting, and almsgiving all impact our health. In the Gospel of Matthew chapter 6, versus 5, 16, and 3, Jesus calls his listeners to prayer, fasting, and almsgiving: "When you pray, do not be like the hypocrites ...when you fast, do not look gloomy...when you give alms, do not let your left hand know what your right is doing." Meditation (prayer) significantly benefits overall well-being and blood pressure control. Fasting is well recognized for its benefits on various bodily functions, including insulin resistance and longevity. Almsgiving has many facets, but "giving of oneself" enhances self-purpose and helps focus on life's purpose, which is essential to emotional health and longevity. The opportunity of a physician to introduce these concepts during office and hospital visits can allow for a more harmonious relationship between the patient and the doctor. It would be misleading to suggest that all my patients embrace these concepts. Still, I also believe that physicians have a unique opportunity to introduce or expand on the healing potential of spirituality.

Interestingly, many recent studies on spirituality in medicine have been related to ICU patients. Cardiologist Randolph Byrd was one of the earliest investigators to identify a beneficial effect of prayer by others on outcomes in hospitalized ICU patients. A subsequent study from the *Archives of Internal Medicine* in 1999 yielded a similar result. ICU patients who were receiving daily prayer from a prayer group had better outcome scores when compared to a control group of patients. One additional (and often quoted) trial suggested that praying for postcoronary bypass patients was not associated with overall benefit. However, the caveat in this trial was the very unusual finding that approximately 50 percent of participants in each group had an unacceptable postoperative complication rate of about 50 percent.

Prayer also appears to have a therapeutic effect on overall health and long-term well-being. Prayer acts as a form of meditation. Cognitive function and reduction in dementia seem to be linked to meditative practice. Group prayer and church attendance have been linked to a more healthy and happy life when measured against other covariables of health analysis. In general, there appears to be a common theme that prayers help both the "pray-ers" and the recipients of those prayers.

In one intriguing study that analyzed obituary information, the benefits of spiritual engagement and participation in religious services appear to prolong life by 5.5–9.5 years. This reduction in mortality far exceeds the benefit of statin therapy in the primary prevention of cardiovascular disease and death. This remarkable statistic adds to the growing evidence that lifestyle "treatments" to reduce the risk of developing heart disease appear superior to most drug therapies. With this knowledge, why isn't spirituality more at the forefront of direct medical care?

Unfortunately, most physicians have not acknowledged that "unconventional" approaches to care can significantly reduce the detrimental impact of cardiovascular disease. Prevailing attitudes vary from dismissive to aggressive condemnation. The current politically correct environment makes many physicians hesitant to embrace these approaches to patient care. This is both sad and disappointing. This humanistic approach should be adopted and advanced rather than actively suppressed.

Physicians and Their Spirituality

I want patients to understand that doctors generally don't discuss spirituality because they do not want to offend their patients. But doctors are not necessarily nonspiritual. Rather, many physicians feel uncomfortable discussing these issues with their patients. In that regard, I offer the option for patients to be more open with their healthcare providers regarding their interest, concern, and willingness to help their doctor become more engaged with their spirituality. It is an opportunity for the patient to "help" doctors to be more aware of the physical and spiritual needs of each patient under their care.

There appears to be a keen interest on the part of patients to discuss and incorporate spirituality into consultations with their physicians. In addition, a large primary care physician study revealed that over 90 percent of physicians considered prayer an essential component of their treatment approach, but less than half incorporated it into their practices. This dichotomy is significant in that physicians likely feel the reluctance to impose a sense of their spirituality on a patient encounter. In my estimation, this is a mistake. Doctors also acknowledge that it is essential to discuss healthy diet patterns. Yet very few take the time to counsel the patient because of time constraints or limited knowledge. We all have good intentions but often fail to follow through with the necessary treatment.

The exact methodology that improves clinical outcomes is not entirely understood, but the results suggest that recovery generally tends to be enhanced when patients receive prayer. The inability of researchers to provide a clear cause-and-effect relationship based on current scientific methodology has resulted in a negative approach to reporting and accepting such studies. One must read the comment sections of journals to realize the negative attitude that prevails when these studies are published. This negativity is typical in the scientific world when studies raise questions that challenge the currently accepted theories and ideologies in medicine. The Cochrane website (www.cochrane.org) is replete with examples of previously held concepts and "scientifically based" practice patterns that have been debunked.

The willingness of a physician to reveal a spiritual openness in patient care shows a nonscientific but compassionate approach that can be embraced, ignored, or rejected by the patient. Fear of being spurned for choosing this methodology may prevent many physicians from revealing their spiritual beliefs. Still, I believe that it is a mistake for physicians to avoid the fear of rejection at the expense of spiritual nurturing. One of the greatest humanitarians in our lifetime, Mother Teresa, directly addressed this issue when she said that the poverty of the West is, *"not only a poverty of loneliness but also of spirituality. There's a hunger for love, as there is a hunger for God."*

Yet as discussed earlier, revealing spirituality, and discussing its benefits on health is not the norm. So where does this now leave us as we try to understand spirituality's role in delivering medical care? My perspective is simple and direct: Physicians should embrace it and attempt to merge our healthcare delivery's physical and metaphysical components. Physicians need to acknowledge that every patient has unique spiritual beliefs, and healthcare providers need to show understanding and withhold judgment no matter how their beliefs might differ from the patients'.

In Christianity, Jesus is the model physician. His healing of the infirm occurred through faith. He did not say that He was the reason for the cure. Faith was the reason (Luke 18: 35–43). This tenet is fundamental in our relationship with patients. We must appeal to faith that their illness is treatable and curable. We must provide hope. I don't imply false hope or unrealistic expectations, but true hope in treatment and potential cure. We must do these things from a perspective of love for our fellow man. This is what the great physicians understood. We cannot simply be automatons that use a "best practices" method to treat an illness. We must embrace the whole person, including the metaphysical qualities within each of us.

Perhaps we, as physicians, are meant for an even higher calling: evangelization. We live in a world that increasingly ignores God's presence and importance in society. In this world, the absence of God has led to a loss of spirituality. It is self-evident that each woman and man is both a physical and a spiritual being.

Disconnection of the spiritual component leads to a blurring of the borders between good and evil and disengages the meaning and purpose of life. God creates us to love. Love is the antidote to corruption, and we must see that love in others through the vision of God. As physicians, we can reestablish faith in God just as Jesus restored sight to the blind beggar in Jericho. We must understand the symbiotic relationship between physical and spiritual treatment of the sick. It is our calling. We must not ignore our duty.

Pope Benedict XVI's words may help emphasize the importance of spirituality in Western society: "One of the great and essential tasks of our evangelization is, as far as we can, to establish habitats of faith and, above all, to find and recognize them."

Ultimately, we physicians and our patients may be best served if we collectively choose to create our own "habitats" to provide the ideal environment for healing. It may also assuage the anxiety and hesitancy of physicians and other healthcare providers if patients were willing to introduce this concept of spirituality into their office and hospital discussions. This approach could present a change in basic assumptions in the patient-doctor relationship and allow both parties to express their spiritual beliefs and treat health issues more comfortably. The transition will not be easy. Studies confirm that it goes against the general comfort level of physicians.

However, it is a worthy and honorable approach. As providers, we must be assured that we are successful in our ability to satisfy the desires of our patients. We cannot change if we are unwilling to open our minds and hearts to the needs of those who trust us. Sometimes, it is the patient who becomes the conduit for this change. Physicians are also human beings and prone to our insecurities and weaknesses. We could genuinely benefit from the introduction of spirituality into our lives. In a certain way, the patient becomes the healer through this interaction. It will not be easy. I am a pragmatist, but I also love challenges. It may be like swimming against the current when introducing these options, but I invite everyone to plunge with me. Let us begin this journey together and see where the story ends!

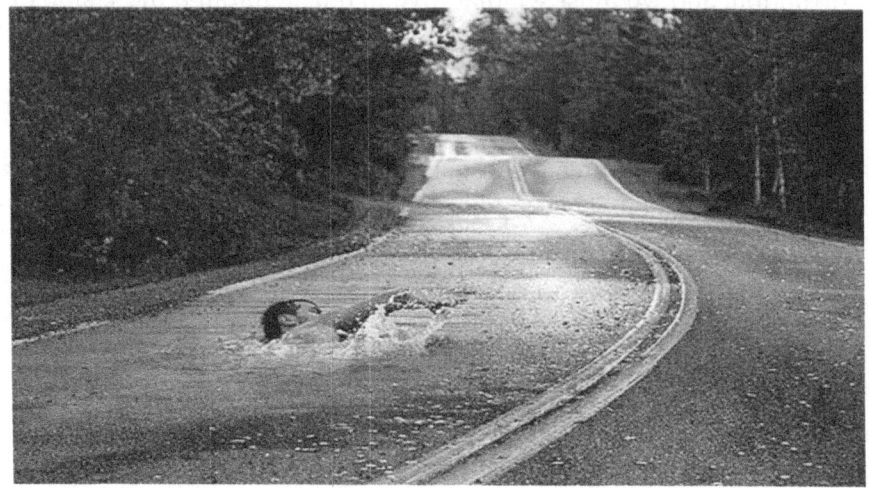

<u>Takeaways</u>

1. Humans are physical and spiritual beings, and patients are open to a spiritual approach to their healthcare even when physicians are hesitant.
2. Multiple scientific studies have identified prayer as a beneficial tool in the healing process.
3. In a world where God is no longer a priority in daily life, physicians can play a vital role in promoting virtue and evangelization in the service of their patients.
4. Healing is a complex process, and interlacing a physical and spiritual approach can provide immeasurable rewards to patients and healthcare workers.

Chapter 9

The Best Diet

One of the most frequent questions patients ask me is what they should eat. I do not intend to write an extensive thesis on this topic anytime soon—volumes of internet material and innumerable books cover this topic in exhaustive detail. However, I hope that this chapter will assist you in identifying important concepts that will guide you toward a successful long-term nutritional plan.

Before I start, let me offer some of my reading favorites for individuals who want to understand the basic dietary philosophy that I favor. I generally caution against oversaturating individuals with too much information and books. At present, the following books are what I consider a great foundation of information that very much aligns with my dietary recommendations. Although they have different approaches to the same problems that we face today, they offer simple directions and are considered (in my opinion) to have authoritative credentials.

- *The Pioppi Diet* by Dr. Aseem Malholtra
- *Food: What the Heck Should I Eat?* by Dr. Mark Hyman
- *Fat Chance* by Dr. Robert Lustig

- *Deep Nutrition: Why Your Genes Need Traditional Food* by Dr. Catherine Shanahan

Two other references that I would suggest including the following:

- *The End of Alzheimer's* by Dr. Dale Bredesen includes nutrition guidelines for dementia prevention and reversal.
- *MIND DIET for Beginners* by Kelli McGrane, MS, RD

    I grew up in an era when the nutritional guidelines were primarily based on a food pyramid created in 1977 by a political assistant with no nutritional training or health expertise. Government guidelines have occasionally been modified since that time but are still heavily influenced by the food industry and political lobbyists. In addition, societies such as the American Heart Association (AHA) and the American Cancer Society (ACS) have significant conflicts of interest. These influential bodies receive substantial financial support from different food industries when they permit the AHA or ACS logo to be printed on foods that would otherwise be considered toxic or unhealthy. We are also bombarded by advertisements and "documentaries" that provide limited or skewed data and half-truths. It is no wonder that individuals are more confused today than ever.

    When reading about nutrition, it's common to find that many authors favor only one magical diet that promises to transform everyone into an incredibly healthy specimen. Unfortunately, you'll only be successful if you strictly adhere to their guidelines for the rest of your life. So many people are so frustrated with their poor health or weight issues that they will torture themselves with dieting for months before they get frustrated and return to their previous favorite foods. This story is repeated nearly daily in my clinic and is both sad and revealing. Patients frequently recognize their poor nutritional choices but cannot generate the willpower or the endurance to overcome these poor habits.

To top it off, many don't even know or understand what they should eat because of all the conflicting messages. There seems to be an ongoing war among well-known "experts" in the diet field. This battle is both confusing and perhaps self-serving. The plant-based experts insist that their diet is ideal, while the meat-based experts insist that their diet is optimum for health. There are low-fat enthusiasts and high-fat advocates. There are low-carbohydrate and high-carbohydrate enthusiasts. It is no wonder that patients get confused and frustrated. There seems to be no compromise among the various camps, and this confusion and dogmatic approach do not benefit the individual trying to optimize their health.

Too often, physicians and other healthcare workers provide standard dietary recommendations such as the Mediterranean diet, the ketogenic diet, or a vegan diet. While I have attempted to keep an open mind while exploring the extensive literature on diet and health, I have found that despite my critics' protests, there is no one "ideal" heart-healthy diet. After caring for thousands of patients over the past many years, I recognize that most people strongly prefer food that tastes good and that they are comfortable with.

I have also come to the hard realization that a physician can rarely convince a patient to radically change their dietary habits if that individual fails to recognize the harm their nutritional choices are doing to their health. My patients are adults who can make their own decisions, even if the long-term consequences of their poor choices are harmful. I often remind them that my staff and I have a shared interest in their long-term health—we are an "accountability office" that wants to see them succeed. Patients will not be chastised or belittled if they fail to meet our expectations, but they can expect honest and direct feedback. We want them to live long, healthy, and happy lives.

Basic Tenets

So, what are we to do with all this conflicting information? There is no one best diet, but there are basic dietary truths.

Humans are omnivores:

We can eat and digest various foods, including meat and plants. We are not exclusively herbivores because humans cannot survive on plants alone without supplementation of vitamin B12, vitamin D, and vitamin A. Omega-3 fatty acids are necessary for survival.

Vegans can obtain adequate vitamin D, vitamin A, and omega-3 fatty acids from plant sources, but it may require careful planning and supplementation to ensure optimal intake. Consultation with a registered dietitian or healthcare provider may be beneficial to ensure a well-planned vegan diet.

While the body naturally produces vitamin D when the skin is exposed to sunlight, we need additional vitamin D from meat. Vegans can get vitamin D from fortified foods such as plant-based milk, orange juice, breakfast cereals, and mushrooms exposed to UV light. A vitamin D supplement may also be necessary, especially during the winter months or if sun exposure is limited.

Vitamin A is essential for vision, immune function, and skin health. While animal foods are the richest sources of vitamin A, vegans can obtain it from plant-based sources such as sweet potatoes, carrots, spinach, and pumpkin. With that said, be aware that plant-based sources of vitamin A contain carotenoids, which the body must convert into active vitamin A. Some people may have difficulty with this conversion and may require a supplement or fortified foods.

Omega-3 fatty acids are essential for heart and brain health. While fatty fish is a rich source of omega-3s, vegans can obtain them from plant-based sources such as flaxseed, chia seeds, hemp seeds, and walnuts. However, these sources primarily provide alpha-linolenic acid (ALA), which the body must convert into the more biologically active forms of omega-3s, EPA and DHA. It may be difficult for some people to convert ALA to EPA and DHA efficiently, and they may need to consider taking an algae-based supplement, which is a vegan source of EPA and DHA.

So, yes, a predominantly plant-based diet can benefit long-term heart health, but I am not convinced that a vegan diet is necessary. Despite its many advantages, most of my patients need help adhering to a vegan lifestyle. Interestingly, we can survive on a carnivore (meat only) diet if we consume raw or organ meats. The battles between plant and meat warriors are mainly unnecessary, as we need both.

Eat more white meat and less red meat:

Meat consumption, especially red meat, is controversial to many experts who write about optimum diet guidelines. But small amounts of red meat (2–3 portions/week) are not harmful and provide valuable nutrients, including iron and essential vitamins. Modest cuts of white meat (poultry and pork) are also quite acceptable, although I avoid pork because of parasite concerns. The difference in fat concentration between white and dark poultry is relatively tiny, so enjoy what you prefer.

Fish is abundant in healthy omega-3 fats and is an excellent addition to your diet. Salmon and cod are good choices and should ideally be wild caught rather than farmed. Wild-caught salmon is generally considered more nutritious than farmed salmon because it contains higher omega-3 fatty acids, vitamin D, and vitamin B12 levels. Wild salmon feed on a natural diet, which includes small fish and algae, while farmed salmon are often fed a diet of grain, soy, and other feed ingredients. Farmed salmon may also contain higher contaminants such as PCBs and dioxins, found in their feed and can accumulate in their flesh. Mercury contamination is a concern for all fish, especially deeper-water fish such as swordfish, bigeye tuna, orange roughy, and Chilean sea bass. Moderation is critical, as heavy metals in fish can be harmful. Selenium-rich foods such as avocado, spinach, and brown rice can counteract mercury toxicity and are simple to add to a lunch or dinner meal.

Whole foods are best:

If you can only carry away one crucial message for long-term dietary health, it is this: consume a whole-food diet. Whole foods are minimally processed foods free of chemical additives and retaining all their natural nutrients and fiber. Whole foods are better than processed foods, a mix of refined, unhealthy ingredients. Processed foods contain various ingredients that can cause underlying inflammation and harm. The food industry primarily focuses on taste and marketing to increase profit and ensure ongoing product use, with little concern for health or nutritional content. Sugar is addictive to the human brain, and processed foods take advantage of this fact with various simple sugars added for flavoring. High fructose corn syrup is toxic to our health, but this ingredient is abundant in many boxed, bagged, and canned products. There is also evidence that products that contain high fructose corn syrup have unacceptable levels of mercury. Stay away from processed foods as much as possible, and your health will improve.

An apple and an egg are whole foods. A box of tasty cereal is not. Most breads are not. Homemade bread made with whole grain flour and minimal processing can still be considered whole food, as it retains the natural nutrients and fiber of the grains used.

However, it's important to note that not all homemade breads are whole foods. Some recipes may use refined flours or other processed ingredients that can reduce their overall nutritional value. A few store-bought breads are also whole. Ezekiel bread, in particular, is made with sprouted whole grains, legumes, and seeds, which are ground into a dough and baked into bread. The sprouting process can increase the availability of nutrients and make the bread easier to digest for some individuals.

Additionally, the portion size and accompanying toppings or spreads can also affect the healthfulness of the bread. Opt for Ezekiel and homemade bread made with whole grain flour and enjoy them in moderation as part of a balanced diet.

Eat organic:

I believe that organic is always the better option, even when the higher cost may pose a financial challenge. You and your body are worth it. But whether my belief is true is a complex and debated topic. Organic foods are produced without synthetic pesticides, fertilizers, and genetically modified organisms (GMOs). They also adhere to specific standards regarding animal welfare and environmental sustainability. I always choose organic foods because pesticides in some nonorganic foods can have a detrimental effect on the gut flora and can enhance inflammation.

Follow the rule of moderation:

Limit calories, avoid excesses in any food group, and limit alcohol and other high-calorie drinks.

Eat fruit in moderation:

I often hear my patients say that they eat an abundance of fruit. There is no question that fruit is generally healthy, but many fruits have a high amount of fructose, and excess fructose may not be suitable for the liver. Consuming too much fructose can cause nonalcoholic fatty liver disease (NAFLD), characterized by the accumulation of fat in the liver. The amount of fruit that can cause liver issues depends on an individual's diet and lifestyle. Thus, it's best to consume fruit in moderation as part of a balanced diet that includes other healthy foods and limits added sugars, including high fructose corn syrup in processed foods and sugary beverages.

Our brain loves sweet things, and it is only logical to migrate toward fruit when attempting to consume a healthy diet, but I recommend two to three servings of fruit per day. I would also suggest that the choice of fruit includes a lower amount of fructose and a reasonable amount of fiber. Good options include berries (raspberries, blueberries, strawberries, blackberries) and citrus fruits (oranges, grapefruits, lemons, and limes). Other good options include avocado and kiwi for those who like its taste. Finally, apples and bananas are not necessarily low in fructose, but they have a reasonable amount of fiber, and they are very popular fruits to consume. Moderation is the guidepost.

Ensure a good balance of healthy fats, carbohydrates, and proteins:

Nutrients can be generally divided into three groups: carbohydrates, proteins, and fats. Many foods are a combination of these, but one usually predominates in each food.

Carbohydrates. After extensive review and personal clinical experience, I believe that a diet with a lower proportion of carbohydrates is probably the best long-term health approach to follow. This conclusion is based on the importance of insulin and its role in modulating obesity and body fat deposition. As a reminder, insulin facilitates cellular growth and repair, inhibits fat breakdown, and promotes the conversion of glucose to fat. High circulating insulin levels also cause the kidneys to retain sodium, which can increase blood pressure. Maintaining lower baseline insulin levels will lead to better health and longevity. But you do still need some carbs. Vegetables and fruits are the best sources of carbohydrates.

Protein. Protein is also generally healthy in moderation, but a higher intake of protein, especially animal protein, may be linked to insulin resistance and possibly type 2 diabetes. Protein comprises amino acids, broken down and used by the body for various functions, including glucose production in the liver. When protein is consumed in excess, the body can convert some of the amino acids into glucose, increasing blood glucose levels. This increase in blood glucose levels can trigger an insulin response to help move glucose out of the bloodstream and into cells for energy.

Then if the body is exposed to high levels of insulin over time (due to chronic consumption of high-protein diets), it can lead to a state of insulin resistance. Insulin resistance occurs when cells become less responsive to insulin signals, leading to higher insulin levels in the blood to maintain normal blood glucose levels. This can eventually lead to the development of type 2 diabetes.

Additionally, some research has suggested that high protein intake, particularly from animal sources, may increase the production of specific amino acids, like branched-chain amino acids (BCAAs), linked to insulin resistance and type 2 diabetes.

Still, moderate consumption of animal protein does not appear to be harmful. Animal protein can be a good source of fat and protein. Plant protein appears to improve insulin sensitivity and is an excellent protein source for higher-risk individuals. So, if you need more protein and don't want to eat meat, plants can be utilized, but vitamin supplementation will be needed.

One caveat regarding protein intake needs to be addressed. As we age, loss of muscle mass develops. This loss is called sarcopenia and can have adverse effects on longevity. It is now advisable for individuals over the age of sixty to increase their daily protein intake to 1.5–2.0 grams per kilogram to offset this issue. Weightlifting is another mechanism to slow or reverse sarcopenia. Protein intake in patients with kidney disease needs to be adjusted and requires discussion with your healthcare provider before increasing daily protein consumption.

Fats. Many of us grew up in an era when fat was considered unhealthy. This long-held premise has been largely disproved except for the issue of trans fats. High consumption of saturated fats found in red meat, eggs, and whole dairy products is associated with increased total cholesterol levels but has not been linked to an increased risk of heart attacks. This ongoing controversy is based on older, faulty studies that were poorly controlled and reported. Higher saturated fat consumption is associated with a rise in HDL without a consistent increase in the small, dense LDL particles linked to CAD. Unsaturated fats (mono- and polyunsaturated) found in fish, nuts, olive oil, and avocado are considered "good" fats and should be part of a regular dietary regimen.

Limit sodium:

While sodium is an essential nutrient our bodies need to function properly, higher sodium consumption can harm our health. The recommended daily sodium intake is 2300 mg or less, about one teaspoon of salt. However, many people consume more sodium than this regularly, which can lead to health problems.

Higher sodium consumption has been linked to high blood pressure, a major risk factor for heart disease, stroke, and other health issues. Too much sodium can also increase the risk of kidney disease, osteoporosis, and stomach cancer.

It's important to note that not all sources of sodium are the same. Sodium from whole foods like vegetables, fruits, and unprocessed meats is typically not a concern for most people. It's the sodium that is added to processed foods and restaurant meals that can contribute to higher sodium intake. To reduce sodium intake, choose fresh, whole foods as much as possible and limit the intake of processed foods and restaurant meals, which can be high in sodium. It is also important to remember that excess sweating and some diuretics can deplete total body sodium. Severe restriction can be very detrimental in these situations and should be periodically monitored by your doctor.

Avoid inflammatory foods whenever possible:

Processed foods, highly refined sugars, products that include high fructose corn syrup, trans fats, and most fried foods fit into this category. While alcohol in small to moderate amounts may have an anti-inflammatory effect, higher consumption of alcohol can cause inflammation of the gut. Please keep in mind, however, that regular, moderate alcohol use does not offset a bad diet. In other words, drinking alcohol under the assumption that it is healthy is misdirected. Alcohol has few medicinal benefits, despite what you may have heard to the contrary.

Pay attention to foods that commonly cause allergies:

If you are allergic, these foods also promote inflammation. The frequency of food allergies is increasing, and one in ten adults is reported to have either a minor or severe food allergy. The most common food allergens include (in order): cow's milk, peanuts, tree nuts (cashews, almonds, walnuts), fish, eggs, wheat, soy, and sesame. In addition, it could be a subtle sign of a food allergy if you have been experiencing chronic gut, brain, or joint issues. For this reason, it is also essential to read labels if you choose to consume processed foods. Finally, gluten sensitivity can be a real issue for some people, and it is remarkable how prevalent gluten is in different foods. There is no definite evidence, however, that gluten-free is a better long-term choice when you have no apparent gluten intolerance.

Consume foods that have both anti-inflammatory and antioxidant benefits:

There are many to choose from. Some of the easiest to incorporate into your weekly diet include:

- berries (blueberries, raspberries, blackberries, and strawberries)
- green leafy vegetables (kale, spinach)
- Broccoli
- fatty fish (salmon, bluefin tuna, sardines)
- nuts (walnuts, Brazil nuts)
- Avocado
- olive (and avocado) oil
- Tomatoes
- dark chocolate (70 percent)

Certain herbs and spices also provide anti-inflammatory and antioxidant benefits, including turmeric, ginger, cinnamon, garlic, black pepper, oregano, and parsley. Unsweetened green tea and coffee also appear to have anti-inflammatory and antioxidant benefits.

It's OK to "Cheat"

It is quite acceptable to cheat occasionally. As we move toward more nutritious food choices, many tend to set unreasonable expectations regarding options and restrictions, eradicating all their favorite foods. So, the idea is to reduce rather than eliminate what is unhealthy. Please remember that food is an essential part of life and should also be enjoyable. Meals should be shared and celebrated communally with family and friends. Food provides cultural and social opportunities that are part of our human fabric, and eating should not be a painful or joyless experience.

Self-discipline is challenging for everyone, so I expect everyone to occasionally falter and give in to a food temptation. A strategy to limit these "hiccups" is very achievable. If you love pizza, try to eat it in limited quantities once every two to three weeks, rather than every Friday night with a few beers. I have personally found that giving myself these small rewards can control my desire for some of my favorite unhealthy foods without destroying my long-term healthy eating goals. I do not believe that you must forever eliminate all poor food choices. Become the master of your diet, and don't let it control you. Life is much too short, and an abundance of great foods is awaiting your enjoyment!

Takeaways

1. There is no perfect diet, but eating unprocessed, whole foods and an organic diet with a smaller overall calorie intake is a good start.
2. Contrary to the previous teaching, processed foods and sugary foods rather than "bad fats" lead to more chronic diseases.
3. Refined carbohydrates are purveyors of many diseases, including diabetes and cardiovascular disease. Therefore, processed foods are the enemy of good health and should be avoided at all costs.
4. Saturated fats do not appear to be as harmful as previously thought. Moderate red meat and egg intake is not conclusively linked to greater cardiovascular risk.
5. Choosing foods with anti-inflammatory and antioxidant components enhances long-term health.
6. Food consumption should be enjoyable, and it should be a shared experience with others. So don't worry about occasional unhealthy choices.

Afterword

Some concluding thoughts. Today, we live in a politically charged world with an ongoing acrimonious debate about whether healthcare is a right or a privilege. As someone immersed in healthcare delivery for more than half my life, I feel that the wrong issue is being debated. Healthcare may or may not be a fundamental right, but good health is a precious commodity that can't be purchased or sold. No medical talisman can magically change lousy health to good health, and patient cooperation (or lack thereof) means that making real health improvements can be very difficult. Consider the fact that over 50% of people over the age of 65 are taking four or more prescription drugs daily, and 40% of individuals in the 18-29 age group are taking at least one prescription daily. This dependence on prescription medicines is very concerning to me. Throughout my medical career, I (and many others) discovered that more is not necessarily better, and less is probably the answer in most circumstances. We seem to be moving in the wrong direction based on our dependence on so many medications.

Voltaire famously stated: *"The art of medicine consists of amusing the patient while nature cures the disease."* In many ways, this is true if no harm is done during the healing process. However, a more aggressive testing and intervention approach is the norm. Sadly, recent data from Dr. Marty Makary suggests that medical errors are now the third leading cause of death. Imaging studies have revealed that over 50% of post-coronary bypass patients have new brain lesions after surgery, and up to one-third of these patients will demonstrate cognitive decline after three years. Yet, patients are still referred for surgery without fully understanding the short and long-term consequences of their treatment. Patients still undergo angioplasty and stent procedures in the hope that it will help them to prolong life and avoid a heart attack. Recent medical studies confirm that medical treatment can be equally effective in most patients. We know that ultra-processed foods lead to weight gain, but there is limited governmental action to restrict these products. Avoidance of social media for as little as one week can significantly lower anxiety and depression, but we continue to scroll and consume the latest information at an alarming rate. We are bombarded with information that is often contradictory regarding medical treatments, and it is no wonder we are confused and frustrated. Coupled with a medical profession that is too busy and the onslaught of marketing ploys from pharmaceutical and device companies, it is no wonder that wellness is declining despite an explosion in costs. This tug of war is not sustainable unless there is a change in the paradigm of healthcare delivery, and it will take cooperation by everyone to make this happen.

By way of example, two medical conditions have been targeted by the pharmaceutical industry since I started writing this book: Dementia and Obesity. Alzheimer's disease is the most common type of dementia and is associated with shrinkage and dysfunction of an area of the brain known as the hippocampus. Dementia is the leading medical condition feared by individuals over the age of 65. Aducanumab is a monoclonal antibody that targets an amyloid beta protein that accumulates in the hippocampus region in patients with early dementia. The drug is only marginally effective and has significant side effects. It slowed the cognitive decline in about 20% of patients but did not reverse the mental deterioration. It must be given intravenously and costs over $50,000 per year. It was approved by the FDA even though 10 of the 11 members of the medical advisory panel voted against its approval. Requests for insurance and Medicare approval were overwhelming once the drug became available. In contrast, a regular aerobic exercise program has been shown to enhance the size of the hippocampus and improve overall memory. Regular exercise in older patients with cognitive decline has been associated with stabilizing and reversing memory impairment. The logical approach to enhance health and improve outcomes in treating cognitive decline is to focus on exercise programs for older adults. This would provide better overall health benefits at a fraction of the cost, but we don't see this information being promoted or widely encouraged. Why not?

Wegovy is a drug that was initially approved for the treatment of Diabetes. It is a manufactured peptide that mimics a satiety hormone known as GLP-1. It requires a weekly injection to maintain efficacy. GLP-1 is primarily produced in the intestinal wall and diminishes hunger while increasing insulin secretion. It has a dual effect of reducing appetite and reducing blood sugar. It is costly ($1400/month) and is not covered by most insurance companies when primarily used as a weight loss agent. A recently completed study utilizing Wegovy injections glowingly reported a 20% relative risk reduction of non-fatal heart attacks and a 7% relative reduction of strokes at three years compared to those patients who did not receive the injection. Immediate calls for Medicare and insurance coverage for Wegovy for cardiac patients have ensued. What is buried in the fine print, however, is that the more critical statistic called absolute risk reduction was only 1.5%. Translated differently, approximately 99 out of 100 patients who took the drug for three years experienced no cardiovascular benefit. In addition, the side effects of the drug are not insignificant. Loss of muscle mass and decreased bone density can occur. Both issues are independently associated with shortened survival. Nausea, vomiting, and diarrhea are common in treated patients and likely contributed to the reported dropout rate of 17% among treated patients. Wegovy results in weight loss, but weight gain returns in many patients when the drug is discontinued. Does this mean that Wegovy is a lifetime medicine? A 50-year-old woman would accrue a 30-year cost of more than $500,000. During this time, she will likely suffer from chronic nausea while increasing her risk of debilitating musculoskeletal issues due to loss of muscle mass and bone density.

In both examples above, an alternative option focused on lifestyle modification, such as regular exercise, reduced carbohydrate intake, and time-restricted eating, could be much better tolerated and effective long-term. The advantages of dramatically reduced healthcare costs and enhanced longevity would be additional benefits. One can imagine the diminished need to utilize healthcare dollars if all of us would spend a little more time taking personal responsibility for our well-being. The total cost of these two drugs alone would endanger the solvency of the Medicare system if broadly utilized by the population.

We are entering an exciting but unknown arena in health care with the growth of artificial intelligence (AI). How AI will impact our current healthcare model is still being determined, but will be significant. Will computer-generated diagnosis and treatment plans diminish or eliminate the need for doctors? What will happen to the compassion and the humanistic qualities essential to care? Will AI-generated algorithms become the norm? I think not, but proper quality health care must be a collaborative effort led by the patient rather than the medical community. As individuals, we take responsibility for our finances, job requirements, and families. We give up that autonomy regarding our health care, which costs us time, money, and years of good health. Personal responsibility for our health will be necessary to avoid financial collapse and rationing. We must refrain from turning over our healthcare to the government and expect quality and access to remain high. We must adhere to good lifestyle habits to maintain health and avoid the healthcare industry's pitfalls.

What is needed? I hope this book has provided information that can be applied to your everyday practice of good health habits. The roadmap does not have to be complex.

Here is a reminder of some of the daily routines that should dramatically enhance your longevity:

- Floss and brush your teeth at least daily.
- Exercise in moderation 5-6 days each week.
- Lift weights 2-3 days a week.
- Eat healthy. Avoid processed foods. Fruits, vegetables, and some unprocessed meats are a good start.
- As you age, emphasize protein consumption, with 1.5-2.0 grams of protein/Kg of weight daily.
- Spend time outdoors and get plenty of early morning sunlight.
- Prioritize sleep and get 6-8 hours each night. It is a critical elixir for long-term health.
- Control daily stress and use prayer/meditation daily. It really helps.
- Engage socially as often as allowed. Attend group and religious activities frequently.
- Use targeted Vitamin D3, fish oil, magnesium, and creatine supplements.
- Limit simple carbohydrates and consider intermittent fasting or time-restricted eating.
- Spend more time with loved ones. Learn to laugh more and have fun!

Shakespeare said, *"Our bodies are our gardens – our wills are our gardeners."* If we are proactive and focus on the daily habits noted above, we will accrue a garden of health that will flower and bloom into a beautiful life filled with joy and purpose. You are worthy of these lofty goals. God wants you to share a life filled with good health and great expectations. My hope and desire are that you will succeed beyond all measure. I also pray that your success will make my efforts worthy of His grace.

God bless.

Acknowledgments

In a way, my book mirrors the downtown Chicago buses I once frequented. As I hopped on and off those city vehicles, collecting experiences, I embraced the insights and observations from contributors on this journey. Like the ever-moving urban landscape, I extend my gratitude to those who've shared their wisdom while boarding and those who've departed, shaping the narrative. Each interaction adds to the colorful map of this book's evolution, reminiscent of my days navigating Chicago's bustling streets.

First and foremost, I want to extend my love and gratitude to my beautiful wife, Jeanne, for her patience, insights, and encouragement. She was my partner on that bus for the entire journey, and I will always cherish the love and guidance that she provided.

I am deeply grateful to my children (Kelly, Meggie, Gabby, and Peter) for your love and encouragement. Your patient insights and tolerance of my frequent obtuse questions helped me immensely throughout this journey.

I completed this project with my excellent editor, Katie Chambers. Her thoughtful insights and guidance were invaluable in completing this project. My proofreader, Laura Major, also offered tremendous insights that allowed the bus to continue in the right direction, and I am deeply grateful for the guidance.

To Drs. Mike Collins, Bryan Foy, and Alan Zelinger, I am incredibly grateful for your wonderful friendship and invaluable insights. Thank you for taking the time to review the manuscripts and offer your valuable comments. As accomplished authors, you have all set a high bar I can only wish to achieve.

To all my wonderful patients who have allowed me to care for them throughout the years. You have taught me and guided me throughout my career and helped make me a more compassionate and humbler physician. Thank you for your patience and your love. I will never forget you.

A physician is but a small part of the entire healthcare system. I am eternally grateful for the outstanding physicians, nurses, administrative staff, and other medical coworkers who have made this journey enjoyable. Even though we doctors think that we are driving the bus, we are backseat passengers who rely entirely on the interaction and help of others. Thank you for your assistance in this incredible medical journey that I have enjoyed.

This book would never have been written without the love and guidance of my wonderful parents. Gene and Rosemary Diamond joined together to create and direct that magical bus filled with all my brothers and sisters. I miss them dearly, but I feel their presence and unwavering love whenever I write.

Finally, I give the highest honor and gratitude to a loving and forgiving God for the gifts he has bestowed on all of us. I am humbled daily by His grace and his guidance. His love profoundly inspires me, and I pray that I have given all glory to Him with this book. I offer it to Him as my small labor of love to all His creation.

A Note to Physicians

As physicians, we are deeply privileged to help our patients overcome their illnesses and improve their overall well-being. While clinical research can provide us with valuable insights, clinical expertise and common sense are essential ingredients in our ability to deliver quality care.

We understand that our patients may desire quick fixes, but we believe in promoting healthy habits like proper nutrition and regular exercise, which can have valuable long-term benefits. Even when faced with difficult cases, such as stable angina, we desire to explore all treatment options to find the best possible solution for our patients rather than relying on a quick fix.

We feel grateful for every small victory we achieve during our work, whether it's successfully treating a heart attack, removing an infected appendix, or helping a patient manage their chronic medical condition. While it can be challenging to work with patients who continue to engage in unhealthy behaviors, we remain dedicated to their well-being, and we are committed to work tirelessly to help them make positive changes.

Although the medical profession can be demanding, we find fulfillment in the positive impact we make on people's lives. We recognize the risk of burnout, but we remain committed to our patients and cherish the privilege of being able to help them lead healthier, happier lives.

Medical doctors belong to a results-driven profession. We want our patients to get better. When I would cut my lawn in the dwindling summer days after work, I truly believed that I was reaching for a final vestige of satisfaction in my day that I could visibly recognize. Seeing the clean lines of the mower on my freshly cut lawn was a visual reminder that I had accomplished a task that was well done and completed. It is no different with the care of patients. We want to achieve the gratification of providing good healthcare even when the results take longer, and the "lines" are somewhat distorted. I have realized that patience is necessary, and persistence is key. As doctors, we need to extend more empathy toward our patients as they struggle to overcome health issues built up over a lifetime of poor habits and guidance. We need to act like copilots that safely and calmly guide our patients to their successful health destination.

A Note to Patients

We have all faced dilemmas in our lives, and we have all faced challenges. Some health challenges can be insurmountable. Still, they should never stop us from continually climbing our personal health mountain. We cannot succumb to a natural inclination of indifference and laziness. We need to joyfully embrace the opportunity to appreciate the proper view of all that this wonderful life has to offer. Good health is worth the effort it takes to achieve. Nothing can replace the future joy of playing basketball with your grandchildren or long walks with friends. Imagine the joy of taking cruises with family and experiencing the energy to play pickleball regularly. See yourself gardening, coaching youth sports, or enjoying an outdoor summer concert. All these pleasures await you when you make that firm commitment to begin a healthy lifestyle. It is never too late to jump on the health bandwagon and join the party. Significant joy awaits you.

I frequently remind my recalcitrant patients that their family is interested in keeping them healthy. If they truly love their spouse and children, they must make the change for them!

This book is a call to arms for all the patients I have been blessed to serve. I yearn for your good health! I want your "golden years" to be golden and lined with great happiness and health. Yes, achieving these results takes cooperative effort, hard work, and discipline, but it *is* possible.

In the end, good health remains a privilege and an enormous gift. We physicians want to "richly and abundantly provide entry" into this realm for our patients. We are all brothers and sisters on the same life path. Let us look forward to the day when we can shed our bad habits as we take the road to good health, longevity, and true happiness.

May God bless all of you, and let the journey begin!

Made in the USA
Monee, IL
22 January 2024